DIGITAL HEALTH FOR PRIMARY CARE

This book provides a comprehensive exploration of the role of Digital Health technologies in Primary Care. Discussing the transformative potential of Digital Health solutions and their impact on healthcare delivery within the Primary Care setting, the book offers insights, considers strategies, and shares practical guidance for all Primary Care providers interested in leveraging digital innovations to enhance patient outcomes and optimise care delivery.

Key Features:

- Content specific to and tailored for primary care and family medicine
- Provides expert opinion and thought leadership on key enablers and hindrances of digital technology within health care systems
- Includes concepts of patient and provider co-design of ideal systems and real-world examples of successful integrations of technologies into patient-centred models of care
- Delivers the essential knowledge for practitioners and policy makers to develop and implement digital health innovation and service redesign

Through structured description of the spectrum of existing digital innovations, all applicable within and relevant to Primary Care, this timely new guide will support clinicians, innovators, and policy makers to maximise the opportunities and challenges that these technologies present. This guide will also enable future doctors, whatever their career aspirations, to understand the importance of digital innovation and its applications in health systems and patient-centred care.

About the Editors:

Ana Luisa Neves MD PhD, Clinical Senior Lecturer in Digital Health, Department of Primary Care and Public Health, Imperial College, London, UK; Chair of the WONCA Working Party on eHealth

Liliana Laranjo MD MPH PhD, Associate Professor, Westmead Applied Research Centre, Sydney Medical School, Faculty of Medicine and Health, University of Sydney, Australia; Deputy Chair of the WONCA Working Party on eHealth.

WONCA Family Medicine

About the Series

The WONCA Family Medicine series is a collection of books written by world-wide experts and practitioners of family medicine, in collaboration with The World Organization of Family Doctors (WONCA). WONCA is a not-for-profit organization and was founded in 1972 by member organizations in 18 countries. It has a membership of about 500,000 family doctors in 118 Member Organizations across 131 countries and territories. These Member Organizations represent more than 90% of the world's population.

How To Do Primary Care Educational Research: A Practical Guide

Mehmet Akman, Valerie Wass, Felicity Goodyear-Smith

ICPC-3 International Classification of Primary Care: User Manual and Classification

Kees van Boven and Huib Ten Napel

Family Medicine in the Undergraduate Curriculum: Preparing Medical Students to Work in Evolving Health Care Systems

Valerie Wass, Victor Ng

Anxiety and Depression in Primary Care: International Perspectives

Sherina Mohd-Sidik, Felicity Goodyear-Smith

Core Values in Family Medicine

Anna Stavdal, Johann Agust Sigurdsson, Felicity Goodyear-Smith

Digital Health for Primary Care

Ana Luisa Neves, Liliana Laranjo

Challenges in Primary Mental Health Care

Christos Lionis, Christopher Dowrick

For more information about this series please visit: https://www.crcpress.com/WONCA-Family-Medicine/book-series/WONCA

DIGITAL HEALTH FOR PRIMARY CARE

EDITED BY

Ana Luisa Neves and Liliana Laranjo

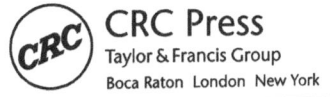

CRC Press
Taylor & Francis Group
Boca Raton London New York

CRC Press is an imprint of the
Taylor & Francis Group, an **informa** business

Designed cover image: Shutterstock

First edition published 2026
by CRC Press
2385 NW Executive Center Drive, Suite 320, Boca Raton FL 33431

and by CRC Press
4 Park Square, Milton Park, Abingdon, Oxon, OX14 4RN

CRC Press is an imprint of Taylor & Francis Group, LLC

ISBN: 978-1-041-00565-0 (hbk)
ISBN: 978-1-041-00563-6 (pbk)
ISBN: 978-1-003-61051-9 (ebk)

DOI: 10.1201/ 9781003610519

Typeset in Minion Pro
by Apex CoVantage, LLC

Contents

Foreword

Digital Health for Primary Care is a much-needed publication from the World Organization of Family Doctors (WONCA) Working Party on eHealth. Digital Health, as defined by the World Health Organization (WHO), encompasses the use of digital technologies to improve health. This broad field includes not only electronic health (eHealth) but also smart, connected devices and emerging technologies such as robotics, big data analytics, and artificial intelligence.

The WONCA Working Party on eHealth is aware of the need to offer a strong evidence-based framework for integrating Digital Health into clinical practice. WONCA, as a global organisation, embraces diversity in uses, opportunities, and challenges of digital innovation. The editors, Ana Luisa Neves and Liliana Laranjo, have brought together an internationally diverse range of authors to combine their knowledge on this important topic for all stakeholders in the delivery of Primary Care.

The resultant book provides a body of knowledge that supports family doctors to embrace digital innovation and optimise its use while critically considering its risks and challenges. The book aims to offer a comprehensive and structured description of the digital innovations that are available, applicable, and relevant to Primary Care. It should thus equip healthcare professionals, particularly family doctors, with the knowledge and understanding necessary to navigate and leverage Digital Health technologies effectively.

Digital Health technologies hold transformative potential particularly in Primary Care. The book includes examples of how this is happening. Already, in my country, many family doctors use AI in our consultations to reduce the time spent on comprehensive notetaking. We profit from the added engagement with our individual patients, as we have increased eye contact with them rather than our computer screens.

It is also acknowledged that effective integration of Digital Health in Primary Care requires a unified approach involving all stakeholders, namely, healthcare providers, patients, policymakers, and technology developers. This includes careful consideration of infrastructure, population needs, workforce training, funding, and resource allocation.

In the final chapter, Drs Laranjo, Ares-Blanco, Howe, Randenikumara, and Li conclude that "Ultimately, the future of Primary Care lies in striking a balance between technological progress and the enduring values of trust, compassion, and equity that define the patient-physician relationship."

This book will contribute to improving health systems throughout the world by strengthening and guiding family doctors and their teams in the use of AI and other technologies. This, is turn, will no doubt improve health outcomes and better achieve *"Health for All"*.

Associate Professor Karen M. Flegg
President, World Organization of Family Doctors (WONCA)
Australian National University Rural Clinical School

Preface

Primary Care is the cornerstone of an effective health system. As the first point of contact for most individuals, Primary Care addresses a broad spectrum of health needs, ranging from prevention to early detection and treatment. By fostering long-term relationships, Primary Care providers aim to deliver personalised, preventive, and continuous care. By integrating services across the wider health system, they ensure that care remains cohesive and comprehensive. The impact of Primary Care is backed by research—studies consistently show that countries with a strong Primary Care system experience a lower mortality rate, better chronic disease management, and improved overall population health.

Today, however, Primary Care is under growing pressure. Ageing populations, rising demand, workforce shortages, and fragmented systems are straining its capacity. Digital innovation has promised to help meet these challenges—and its relevance has never been more urgent.

Despite historically slow digital adoption in Primary Care, since 2020, this landscape has shifted dramatically. The COVID-19 pandemic acted as a catalyst for digital transformation by accelerating the adoption of digital tools. Advances in artificial intelligence—now more powerful and accessible than ever—have created further momentum. Importantly, digital innovation has not been confined to the clinical setting. Patients and the public are now ubiquitously using technology to manage their health outside traditional care encounters by tracking symptoms, monitoring conditions, and accessing health information independently, all at their fingertips. This shift offers an opportunity to support patients at the intersection of daily self-management and clinical oversight and to view health as a continuous journey rather than as a series of isolated episodes. Much of the health experience happens outside the formal healthcare system, and digital tools can help us finally begin to bridge this gap.

In lieu of offering a technical manual, this book aims to answer these questions by providing insights into how digital technology is reshaping clinician–patient interactions, impacting outcomes, and transforming the design and delivery of Primary Care. We examine the core technologies that shape the field and assess their influence on key domains of healthcare quality, such as clinical effectiveness, patient-centredness, safety, and equity. We also reflect on the importance of user-centred design, implementation strategies, sustainability in the context of systems thinking, and the future path towards the meaningful integration of technology into the complex jigsaw of healthcare delivery.

We are fully aware that technology will continue to evolve and that many of the specific tools and examples discussed in this book may become outdated or incomplete in the near future. However, we believe that the core concepts explored here, particularly those related to user-centred design, impact assessment, and sustainable implementation and integration, will remain essential. These foundational principles provide a framework for understanding and navigating the digital transformation in Primary Care, irrespective of changes in the actual technologies. Our aim is to offer insights that are adaptable and relevant across settings and over time.

We are deeply grateful to our global network of contributors: their local insights, generosity, and collaborative spirit were instrumental in shaping this narrative.

This book reflects our belief in the principle of "learning globally, acting locally", and our hope is that this work will allow us to build bridges that support positive change. We hope that this book informs, provokes, and inspires action toward a future where Digital Health enables a more connected, compassionate, and effective Primary Care.

The Editors,
Ana Luisa Neves
Liliana Laranjo

About the Editors

Ana Luisa Neves (MD, MSc, PhD) is a Clinical Associate Professor in Digital Health at Imperial College London. Dr Neves is a practicing GP, and currently holds roles as Chair of the Working Party on eHealth of WONCA World and Vice-Chair of the European General Practice Research Network. At Imperial, Dr Neves is Director of the Global Digital Health, leads the Digital Health Theme at the Northwest London NIHR Applied Research Collaboration, and is Co-Lead for the Theme 'New service delivery models' at the Northwest London NIHR Patient Safety Research Collaboration. She also holds a position as Invited Associate Professor at University of Porto. She coordinates multidisciplinary research teams focusing on the design, implementation and evaluation of digital technologies to deliver safer, more effective, and patient-centred care.

Dr. Neves has a Master of Science from University of Porto (Portugal) and a PhD in Clinical Medicine from Imperial College London (UK). During her PhD, she received a PhD studentship from the GABBA Program (Graduate Program in Areas of Basic and Applied Biology), a international PhD program funded by the Portuguese Foundation for Science and Technology. In 2018, Dr. Neves was awarded a WONCA Scholarship, followed by an Athena SWAN Award for Excellence at Imperial College London in 2019. She completed the Global Health Leaders Program at Harvard University in 2022–2023. Dr Neves was appointed as a Visiting Scholar at the Harvard T.H. Chan School of Public Health (2024–2025), as part of her International Fellowship at Ariadne Labs. Dr Neves has more than 6,500 citations, with an h-index of 32.

Liliana Laranjo (MD, MPH, PhD) is an Associate Professor at Sydney Medical School, University of Sydney, where she holds a Sydney Horizon Fellowship. She has a background as a General Practitioner and is Deputy Chair of the World Organization of General Practitioners' (WONCA) eHealth Working Party, as well as Member of the founding International Advisory Board for The Lancet Primary Care. Dr. Laranjo leads the Digital Health Stream at the Westmead Applied Research Centre, an Impact Centre of the University of Sydney, where she coordinates several clinical trials and leads multidisciplinary teams across different fields, from medicine and health to data science and engineering. Her research focuses on leveraging Digital Health to empower and support patients in their health journeys, with the aim of preventing chronic disease at scale in the community.

Dr. Laranjo has a Master of Public Health from Harvard University and a PhD in Medicine (Digital Health) from Lisbon Medical School, Portugal. During her PhD, she received a Junior Clinical Research Award from the Harvard Medical School-Portugal Program. She was a 2022 World Heart Federation Emerging Leader and has been awarded a National Health and Medical Research Council Emerging Leader Investigator Grant (2023–2027) and an Honorary Future Leader Fellowship from the National Heart Foundation (2023–2026) in Australia. Dr. Laranjo's work has received global media attention and has been used to guide research, practice, and policy worldwide. Her field-weighted citation index is 2, meaning her overall number of citations is double the world average in the field.

Contributors

Ahmed Alboksmaty
Institute of Global Health
    Innovation (IGHI)
Department of Surgery and Cancer
Imperial College London
London, United Kingdom

Douglas Aninng Opoku
Department of Epidemiology and
    Biostatistics
School of Public Health
Kwame Nkrumah University of
    Science and Technology
Kumasi, Ghana

Sara Ares-Blanco
Federica Montseny Health Centre
Gerencia Asistencial Atención
    Primaria
Servicio Madrileño de Salud
Madrid, Spain;
Research Network on Chronicity
Primary Care and Health
    Promotion-RICAPPS-(RICORS)
    Spain
Instituto de Investigación Sanitaria
    Gregorio Marañón
Madrid, Spain

Ulrik Bak Kirk
Department of Public Health
Aarhus University
Aarhus, and
Research Unit for General Practice
Aarhus, Denmark

Mariam Beridze
World Health Organization
Country Office Georgia
Data and Digital Health Officer
Tbilisi, Georgia

Jako Burgers
Care and Public Health Research
    Institute
Department of Family Medicine
Maastricht University
Maastricht, The Netherlands

See Chai Carol Chan
Department of Primary Care and
    Public Health
Imperial College London
London, United Kingdom

Niels Chavannes
Department of Public Health and
    Primary Care/National eHealth
    Living Lab
Leiden University Medical Center
Leiden, The Netherlands

Kam Cheong Wong
Westmead Applied Research Centre
Faculty of Medicine and Health
University of Sydney, NSW,
    Australia; Bathurst Rural
    Clinical School
School of Medicine, Western
    Sydney University
NSW, Australia

Jacopo Demurtas
Family Medicine Department
USL Toscana Sud-Est
Grosseto, Italy

Hans Eguia
Family Medicine Clinic
Lægehuset Engdraget
Rudkobing, Denmark

Ana Ferreira
RISE-HEALTH, Department of
    Community Medicine
Information and Health Decision
    Sciences
Faculty of Medicine
University of Porto, Portugal

Tom Freeman
Centre for Studies in Family
    Medicine
Schulich School of Medicine and
    Dentistry
London, Ontario, Canada

Francisca Gaifém
Research Unit for Global Health
Department of Public Health
Aarhus University, Aarhus, Denmark

Avivit Golan Cohen
Faculty of Medical and Health
    Sciences
Tel Aviv University
Tel Aviv, Israel

Raquel Gómez Bravo
Centre Hospitalier Neuro-
    Psychiatrique (CHNP)
Ettelbruck, Luxembourg
Department of Behavioural and
    Cognitive Sciences
University of Luxembourg

Geva Greenfield
Department of Primary Care and
    Public Health
School of Public Health
Imperial College London
London, United Kingdom

Nick Guldemond
Tsinghua University
Research Center for Medical
    Sociology
Beijing, China

Benedict Hayhoe
Department of Primary Care and
    Public Health
School of Public Health
Imperial College London
London, United Kingdom

Boon How Chew
Department of Family Medicine
Faculty of Medicine and Health
    Sciences
Universiti Putra Malaysia
Serdang, Selangor, Malaysia

Amanda Howe
Norwich Medical School
University of East Anglia
Norwich, Norfolk

Cristina Jácome
RISE-HEALTH, Department of
    Community Medicine
Information and Health Decision
    Sciences
Faculty of Medicine
University of Porto, Portugal

Geronimo Jimenez
Department of Public Health and
    Primary Care
Leiden University Medical Center
Leiden, The Netherlands

Marise Kasteleyn
Department of Public Health and
    Primary Care
National eHealth Living Lab
Leiden University Medical Center
Leiden, The Netherlands

Karen Kinder
Working Party on eHealth
WONCA World

Pratyush Kumar
DNB Patna Physician & Diabetes
    Clinic
Patna, Bihar, India

Obed Kwabena Offe Amponsah
Department of Pharmacy Practice
Faculty of Pharmacy and
    Pharmaceutical Sciences
Kwame Nkrumah University of
    Science and Technology
Kumasi, Ghana

Nana Kwame Ayisi-Boateng
University Health Services
Kwame Nkrumah University of
    Science and Technology
Kumasi, Ghana

Liliana Laranjo
Westmead Applied Research
    Centre
Sydney Medical School
Faculty of Medicine and Health
University of Sydney, Sydney,
    Australia

Donald Li
Hong Kong College of Family
    Physicians
Honorary Professor of Family
    Medicine
University of Hong Kong; Chairman
Elderly Commission of
    Hong Kong

Edmond Li
Department of Primary Care and
    Public Health
Imperial College London
London, United Kingdom

Olivia Lounsbury
Nuffield Department of Clinical
    Neurosciences
University of Oxford
Oxford, United Kingdom

Azeem Majeed
Department of Primary Care and
    Public Health
Imperial College London
London, United Kingdom

Nancy Matillya
Department of Family Medicine
Aga Khan University
Dar es Salaam, Tanzania

Ana Luisa Neves
Department of Primary Care and
    Public Health
Imperial College London
London, United Kingdom

Eric Kojo Nsa Oduro
University Hospital
Kwame Nkrumah University of
    Science and Technology
Kumasi, Ghana

Rebecca Payne
North Wales Medical School
Bangor University
Bangor, and Nuffield Department of
    Primary Healthcare Sciences
University of Oxford
Oxford, United Kingdom

Unben Pillay
Africa Telehealth Collaboration (ATC)
United Forum of Family
    Practitioners (UFFP)
Johannesburg, South Africa

Pramendra Prasad
Department of General Practice and
    Emergency Medicine
B.P. Koirala Institute of Health
    Sciences
Dharan, Nepal

Sankha Randenikumara
The Family Health Clinic
Colombo, Sri Lanka

Ana Rita Luz
MTG Research & Development Lab,
    Porto, Portugal

Andree Rochfort
Irish College of GPs
Dublin; Department of General
    Practice
Legal and Forensic Medicine
University College Dublin, Ireland

Bridget L. Ryan
Centre for Studies in Family Medicine
Departments of Family Medicine and
    Epidemiology and Biostatistics
Schulich School of Medicine &
    Dentistry
Western University
London, Canada

Hüsna Sarıca Çevik
Department of Family Medicine
Ankara University School of
    Medicine
Ankara, Türkiye

Melita Sogomonjan
Visiting Lecturer at the Tallinn
    University of Technology
Tallinn, Estonia

Bernardo Sousa-Pinto
MEDCIDS—Department of
    Community Medicine
Information and Health Decision
    Sciences
Faculty of Medicine of the
    University of Porto
Porto, Portugal

Moira Stewart
Centre for Studies in Family
    Medicine
Department of Family Medicine,
    Schulich School of Medicine &
    Dentistry
Western University, London,
    Canada

Paulien Tensen
Department of Public and
    Occupational Health
Amsterdam Public Health,
    Amsterdam UMC location
University of Amsterdam
Amsterdam, The Netherlands

Keith Thompson
Center for Studies in Family
  Medicine
Department of Family Medicine
Schulich School of Medicine and
  Dentistry
Western University
London, Canada

Mehmet Ungan
Department of Family
  Medicine
Ankara University School of
  Medicine
Ankara, Türkiye

Steven van de Vijver
Amsterdam Public Health
Amsterdam UMC location
University of Amsterdam
Amsterdam, The Netherlands

Shlomo Vinker
Faculty of Medical and Health
  Sciences
Tel Aviv University
Tel Aviv, Israel

Mercy Wanjala
Africa Forum for Primary Health
  Care
Nairobi, Kenya

Raluca Zoițanu
Department of Public Health
Babeș-Bolyai University
Cluj-Napoca, Romania

Acronyms and Abbreviations

ADL	Activity of daily living
AI	Artificial intelligence
AI-CDSS	Artificial intelligence-powered clinical decision support systems
CDSS	Clinical decision support systems
COVID-19	Coronavirus disease 2019
DHEF	Digital Health equity framework
DHE	Digital Health equity
DHTs	Digital Health technologies
DSMSTs	Digital self-management support tools
EHDS	European health data space
EHR	Electronic health record
EPHR	Electronic personal health record
EU	European Union
FDA	US Food and Drug Administration
FM	Family medicine
FPM	Family practice model
GDPR	General Data Protection Regulation
GP	General Practitioner
GSMA	Global System for Mobile Communications Association
HIPAA	Health Insurance Portability and Accountability Act
ICTs	Information and communication technologies
ITU	International Telecommunication Union
LLM	Large language model
LMICs	Low- and middle-income countries
MARS	Mobile app rating scale
mHealth	Mobile health applications
ML	Machine learning
NCDs	Non-communicable diseases
NIA	National Institute on Aging
NIMHD	National Institute on Minority Health and Health Disparities
NLP	Natural language processing
PCCM	Patient-centred clinical method
PHC	Primary health care
PHR	Personalised health record

PKB	Patients know best
SDH	Social determinants of health
TCO	Total cost of ownership
WHO	World Health Organization

CHAPTER 1

Understanding Digital Health in Primary Care

See Chai Carol Chan, Jako Burgers, Pramendra Prasad, Mehmet Ungan, Karen Kinder, Azeem Majeed, and Ana Luisa Neves

THE PRIMARY CARE LANDSCAPE: CONTEXT IN GLOBAL HEALTH SYSTEMS

Primary Care forms the cornerstone of effective healthcare delivery worldwide to provide accessible and community-based care.[1] Importantly, it often serves as the first point of contact for individuals with the health system. Unlike secondary or tertiary healthcare, Primary Care addresses a wide range of health needs: it promotes preventive health measures, supports early diagnosis, facilitates treatment for both acute and chronic conditions, and coordinates care when patients require secondary care treatment.[1] Additionally, Primary Care aims to reduce the overall burden on healthcare systems by enabling personalised and continuous care that adapts to individual needs.

Despite its pivotal role, Primary Care systems vary significantly across high-income and low-income settings. There are widely recognised examples of well-established Primary Care systems in high-income countries, with robust resource allocation and comprehensive infrastructures—such as the government-funded National Health Service (NHS) in the United Kingdom (UK) or Australia's Medicare system—that offer publicly funded Primary Care services to ensure essential health services when needed. However, even in high-income countries, challenges related to accessibility and equity

DOI: 10.1201/9781003610519-1

persist. Such barriers can delay treatments, disrupt continuity of care, and cause reliance on emergency services for non-urgent health issues.

In contrast, low- and middle-income countries face more substantial resource constraints that hinder consistent provision of high-quality Primary Care. These barriers include a low density of healthcare professionals, under-resourced medical facilities, limited health infrastructure, and inadequate funding. Furthermore, Primary Care in many of these settings often serves as the only accessible form of healthcare for large segments of the population. To bridge this gap in access, Community Health Worker (CHW) programmes have emerged as innovative strategies. These programmes deploy trained local workers to reach underserved communities to provide essential services such as maternal and child care, vaccination programmes, and health literacy education. In the last decade, the world has been affected by various disasters, conflicts, severe weather events, mass casualty events, the pandemic, and earthquakes—further requiring an appropriate preparedness to cope with both current and emerging challenges in Primary Care delivery.

DEFINITION AND CONCEPT OF DIGITAL HEALTH

The definitions and scope of Digital Health vary across different contexts, reflecting its complexity and diverse applications.

The **World Health Organization (WHO)** defines Digital Health as "the field of knowledge and practice associated with the development and use of digital technologies to improve health".[2] It clarifies that Digital Health expands on the concept of electronic health (eHealth) to include smart, connected devices and emerging technologies such as robotics, big data analytics, and artificial intelligence. The WHO Global Strategy on Digital Health 2020–2025 provides additional nuance to the discussion by emphasising the disruptive potential of digital innovation in healthcare and the growing consensus that its strategic and innovative use can promote universal health coverage. The WHO also emphasises that Digital Health should be developed with principles of transparency, accessibility, scalability, replicability, interoperability, privacy, security, and confidentiality to optimally benefit people in a way that is ethical, safe, equitable, and sustainable.

The **European Commission** highlights the potential of Digital Health to improve access to care, the quality of care, and the efficiency of the health sector. It refers to Digital Health and care as "the tools and services that use information and communication technologies (ICTs) to improve prevention, diagnosis, treatment, monitoring and management of health-related issues".[3] Moving forward, the **European Commission** identifies three key priorities: secure data access and sharing across borders; connecting and sharing health data for research; and citizen empowerment with digital tools.

The **United States Food and Drug Administration (FDA)** reiterates and re-emphasises the potential of Digital Health in improving the ability to both diagnose and treat diseases and to deliver healthcare. It discusses the broad scope of Digital Health, which encompasses "technologies intended for use as a medical product, in a medical product, as companion diagnostics, or as an adjunct to other medical products (devices, drugs, and biologics)".[4] Examples include wearable devices, telehealth and telemedicine, and personalised medicine. Furthermore, Digital Health may be used to develop or study medical products. The **FDA** Digital Health Center of Excellence and its Digital Health Innovation Action Plan were developed to regulate Digital Health tools to ensure that they meet safety and efficacy standards.

These various definitions and perspectives are examples that demonstrate the multifaceted nature of Digital Health. These definitions converge on shared goals, such as enhancing care delivery, improving access, and advancing health outcomes, but they differ in focus. The FDA emphasises regulatory frameworks, the European Commission prioritises innovation and empowerment, and the WHO adopts a global health perspective that highlights equity, ethical implementation, and universal access implications.

Digital Health can be broadly categorised into the three primary areas of **communication technologies**, **diagnostic technologies**, and **management technologies**.[5] All can play a critical role in supporting Primary Care delivery and enhancing patient outcomes. Box 1.1 shows several introductory examples, with further exploration and discussion in Chapter 2.

BOX 1.1   INTRODUCTORY EXAMPLES OF DIGITAL HEALTH TECHNOLOGIES

Communication Technologies

1.1. **Telehealth:** Telehealth refers to the use of digital technologies to deliver healthcare services remotely. This can include virtual consultations (via video or phone calls) and even e-prescriptions or remote access to health records via patient portals.

1.2. **Mobile health applications:** Mobile health applications can support health education, facilitate chronic disease management, and empower patients to monitor their own health.

Diagnostic Technologies

2.1. **Machine learning (ML):** ML can use healthcare data to explain what happened, predict what may happen, or make recommendations on what to subsequently do. By analysing patient data and identifying patterns, these approaches can be used to streamline diagnostic processes and enable earlier interventions for chronic conditions.

Management Technologies
3.1. **Electronic health records (EHRs):** EHRs provide a unified platform for storing and accessing patient data. They enhance care continuity, reduce administrative burdens, and facilitate better coordination among multidisciplinary teams.
3.2. **Wearables:** Devices such as smartwatches and biosensors collect real-time health data and allow patients to monitor conditions between consultations.

EVOLUTION OF DIGITAL HEALTH IN PRIMARY CARE

Digital Health has profoundly transformed the landscape of Primary Care to offer new opportunities for enhanced patient care. Over recent decades, digital adoption has accelerated, especially because of technological advancements, policy incentives, and unprecedented challenges such as the COVID-19 pandemic.[6] Restriction or disruption of routine healthcare, a lack of physicians, the protection of healthcare users/patients/providers, shortages of personal protective equipment, and other pressures on healthcare systems have forced these systems to adapt in response to emerging contemporary challenges, ultimately accelerating Digital Health development.[2]

Digital Health in Primary Care has now shifted from being a futuristic concept to an integral component of care delivery especially during the COVID-19 pandemic and has been shaped by varying global adoption patterns.[7] For example, government-mandated pandemic control measures created the necessity of virtual care and forced telehealth, e-prescriptions, and a range of digital communication tools as the preferred means of use, with health systems globally witnessing exponential growth in their use as part of the emergency response.[8] In the United States (US), telehealth visits surged by over 50% in early 2020 compared to pre-pandemic levels.[9] Similarly, the UK's NHS reported that over 90% of general practice consultations transitioned to phone or video calls during the height of the pandemic.[7]

As part of this digital transition, telemedicine has been suggested not only to improve access to high-quality healthcare but also to decrease infection risk in low- and middle-income countries (LMICs).[10] The rapid shift in adoption of Digital Health has demonstrated its potential for maintaining continuity of care amidst disruption—while exposing important gaps, such as disparities in access to technology and digital literacy. Concerns remain about the correct balance between face-to-face and virtual care services and its implications for the quality, safety, and equity of care. Methodologically robust research, leveraging quantitative, real-world data, alongside user-centric approaches that capture user experiences are critical to address this knowledge gap.

GLOBAL ADOPTION PATTERNS OF DIGITAL HEALTH

While Digital Health adoption has been universal, its pace and scale vary across regions because of differing levels of healthcare infrastructure, policy support, investment, and acceptance. High-income countries have generally embraced Digital Health through substantial investments in health IT infrastructure and regulatory frameworks. For example, Scandinavian countries such as Denmark have integrated EHRs nationwide to enable seamless information exchange and population health monitoring.[11] Middle-income countries like India and Brazil are utilising mobile health (mHealth) solutions to address gaps in access: a prime example is India's Ayushman Bharat Digital Mission to create a unified Digital Health ecosystem.[12] Conversely, low-income countries and resource-limited settings often depend on innovative yet low-cost, frugal technologies. For example, SMS-based health interventions have been used to support maternal health in Sub-Saharan Africa.[13] These patterns highlight a common theme: Digital Health solutions must be tailored to the unique needs and resources of each region.

IMPACT ON QUALITY OF CARE

To assess the impact of Digital Health on Primary Care, whether positively or negatively, a comprehensive framework is needed to oversee all relevant aspects.[14] The analytic framework developed by the Institute of Medicine (IOM) in the US is often used for quality assessment and to explore the potential impact of innovations in healthcare, including digital care. The framework contains six dimensions (Box 1.2).

BOX 1.2   AIMS FOR HEALTHCARE IMPROVEMENT[15]

- **Safety:** avoiding harm to patients from the care that is intended to help them.
- **Effectiveness:** providing services based on scientific knowledge to all who could benefit and refraining from providing services to those not likely to benefit (avoiding underuse and misuse, respectively).

- **Patient-centredness:** providing care that is respectful of and responsive to individual patient preferences, needs, and values and ensuring that patient values guide all clinical decisions.
- **Timeliness:** reducing waiting and sometimes harmful delays for both those who receive and those who give care.
- **Efficiency:** avoiding waste, including waste of equipment, supplies, ideas, and energy.
- **Equity:** providing care that does not vary in quality because of personal characteristics such as gender, ethnicity, geographic location, and socioeconomic status.

Safety is a fundamental priority, aligning with Hippocrates' oath to "first, do no harm". Digital care presents potential risks, particularly in cases where face-to-face interactions may be key, such as acute and palliative care. Ensuring the **effectiveness** of digital care is essential in evaluating its benefits and added value. **Person-centred care** is integral to Digital Health, as individual preferences, needs, and values must be prioritised when implementing digital solutions. **Timeliness** is another key factor, with digital tools offering opportunities to accelerate diagnosis and treatment while reducing waiting times for consultations and referrals. From an **efficiency** perspective, digital care has the potential to lower costs by optimising personnel use, reducing travel, and minimising equipment needs. However, the initial setup and ongoing maintenance of digital technologies also introduce significant financial considerations. Finally, achieving **equitable** digital care remains a challenge. The availability and affordability of digital tools, such as mobile devices, are not universally covered by healthcare plans, and disparities in digital literacy may deepen existing inequities in healthcare access and use. Addressing these challenges is essential to ensure that Digital Health benefits all patients, regardless of their background or resources.[16,17]

Professional Satisfaction

The resources and skills of healthcare professionals vary widely. Moreover, the attitude towards introducing innovations, such as Digital Health, varies from pioneers taking the initiative to laggards reluctant to change their routines and habits. Implementation strategies to change behaviour should include a mix of top-down and bottom-up interventions to ensure professional satisfaction.

This is increasingly important to retain the workforce in Primary Care.[18] Digital healthcare is based on a relationship between providers and consumers, which can thrive only if it benefits both.

Shared Decision-Making

Digital Health solutions are developing in Primary Care, but there is no one-size-fits-all for their use. These solutions depend on the needs and preferences of both patients and their caregivers. For example, in diabetes care, some patients may want to share blood glucose values through shared electronic health records; others may not have the skills, resources, or willingness to do so. Routes to access should be preserved in either case to ensure that digital transformation is not leading to exclusion or underservice to those who need care the most. Clinical practice guidelines can support the conscientious use of Digital Health based on evidence, professional expertise, and patient experiences and preferences, thus promoting person-centred care.[19,20]

DIGITAL PRIMARY CARE: THE WAY FORWARD

Digital Health offers immense potential, but its implementation is not without challenges. Issues such as data privacy, data ownership, interoperability, inequities in access, regulations, and user engagement (from both patients and providers) remain critical aspects to consider.[21] Moreover, any efforts to implement Digital Health solutions must recognise that innovation is more likely to be adopted by—and provide the greatest benefits to—individuals with higher literacy and better access to technology. There is a real risk that digital advancements could deepen existing health disparities. To mitigate this, equity must be prioritised at every stage of digital implementation, from initial design and co-development to ongoing evaluation. Establishing effective feedback loops is essential to prevent the digital divide from widening health inequalities; this requires targeted interventions to promote inclusivity and ensure equitable access for all. Looking ahead, the future of Digital Health in Primary Care must focus on personalisation, integration, and accessibility to maximise its impact. Ensuring the active involvement of Primary Care professionals in the development of these innovations is also crucial in aligning digital solutions with both patient needs and clinical practice.

Digital Health has already reshaped Primary Care and will continue to do so. Although adoption levels differ across regions, the direction of travel is clear—towards a more connected, integrated, and patient-centred system.

KEY MESSAGES

- Digital Health has transformed Primary Care globally through technologies such as telemedicine, AI-driven diagnostics, and wearable devices.
- Adoption of Digital Health varies among high-, middle-, and low-income countries.
- Digital Health has the potential to significantly impact the six dimensions of quality of care—safety, efficiency, equity, timeliness, effectiveness, and patient-centredness.
- Digital Health in Primary Care must overcome barriers such as digital literacy gaps, data security concerns, and resource inequities. Its trajectory should focus on achieving the sustainable, equitable, and efficient integration of emerging technologies.
- Shared decision-making between Primary Care providers and patients is critical for the successful and person-centred adoption of Digital Health technologies in Primary Care.

REFERENCES

1. World Health Organization. *Primary health care.* 2024. Available from: https://www.who.int/health-topics/primary-health-care#tab=tab_1.
2. World Health Organization. *Global strategy on digital health 2020–2025.* Geneva: World Health Organization; 2021. Available from: https://www.who.int/docs/default-source/documents/gs4dhdaa2a9f352b0445bafbc79ca799dce4d.pdf.
3. European Commission, Public Health. *eHealth: digital health and care.* Cited 2024 Dec 16. Available from: https://health.ec.europa.eu/ehealth-digital-health-and-care/overview_en.
4. US Food and Drug Association. *Digital health center of excellence.* 2024. Cited 2024 Dec 16. Available from: https://www.fda.gov/medical-devices/digital-health-center-excellence.
5. World Health Organization. *Digital health platform handbook: building a digital information infrastructure (infostructure) for health.* Geneva: World Health Organization; 2020.
6. Monaghesh E, Hajizadeh A. The role of telehealth during COVID-19 outbreak: a systematic review based on current evidence. *BMC Public Health.* 2020;20(1):1193.
7. Murphy M, Scott LJ, Salisbury C, et al. Implementation of remote consulting in UK Primary Care following the COVID-19 pandemic: a mixed-methods longitudinal study. *Br J Gen Pract.* 2021;71(704):e166–77.
8. Koonin LM, Hoots B, Tsang CA, et al. Trends in the use of telehealth during the emergence of the COVID-19 pandemic—United States, Jan–Mar 2020. *MMWR Morb Mortal Wkly Rep.* 2020;69(43):1595–9.
9. Accenture. *Digital health consumer survey 2020.* Available from: https://www.accenture.com/us-en/insights/health/leaders-make-recent-digital-health-gains-last.
10. McKinsey & Company. *Digital health adoption: the future of healthcare.* Available from: https://www.mckinsey.com/business-functions/mckinsey-digital.
11. Christensen CM, Grossman JH, Hwang J. *The innovator's prescription: a disruptive solution for healthcare.* New York: McGraw-Hill Education; 2009.

12. Ministry of Health and Family Welfare, India. *Ayushman Bharat digital mission.* Available from: https://abdm.gov.in/.

13. Free C, Phillips G, Watson L, et al. The effectiveness of mobile-health technologies to improve health care service delivery processes: a systematic review and meta-analysis. *PLoS Med.* 2013;10(1):e1001363.

14. Neves AL, Burgers J. Digital technologies in Primary Care: implications for patient care and future research. *Eur J Gen Pract.* 2022 Dec;28(1):203–8.

15. Institute of Medicine (US) Committee on Quality of Health Care in America. *Crossing the quality chasm: a new health system for the 21st century.* Washington, DC: National Academies Press; 2001.

16. Chang JE, Lai AY, Gupta A, et al. Rapid transition to telehealth and the digital divide: implications for Primary Care access and equity in a post-COVID era. *Milbank Q.* 2021 Jun;99(2):340–68.

17. Kim H, Xie B. Health literacy in the eHealth era: a systematic review of the literature. *Patient Educ Couns.* 2017 Jun;100(6):1073–82.

18. Bodenheimer T, Sinsky C. From triple to quadruple aim: care of the patient requires care of the provider. *Ann Fam Med.* 2014 Nov–Dec;12(6):573–6.

19. Murad MH, Montori VM, Guyatt GH. Incorporating patient preferences in evidence-based medicine. *JAMA.* 2008 Dec 3;300(21):2483.

20. Greenhalgh T, Misak C, Payne R, et al. Patient involvement in developing clinical guidelines. *BMJ.* 2024 Nov 8;387:q2433. https://doi.org/10.1136/bmj.q2433.

21. Blease C, O'Neill S, Walker J, et al. Sharing clinical notes with patients: a meaningful change in the digital health era. *BMJ.* 2020;371:m3795.

CHAPTER 2

Digital Health Tools for Clinical Practice

Edmond Li, Olivia Lounsbury,
Bernardo Sousa-Pinto, Unben Pillay,
Avivit Golan Cohen,
and Shlomo Vinker

INTRODUCTION

Digital Health technologies are becoming increasingly central to care delivery in most clinical settings, with many benefits. For example, for clinicians, Digital Health technologies can help ease the burden of administrative tasks and free up more time for patient-facing clinical activities. For patients, Digital Health technologies have improved, for example, their access to care across geographies and for complex care needs. There are, however, several implications regarding the use of Digital Health technologies for clinical care, and although they offer significant benefits, they are not without risks. This chapter aims to provide an overview of common Digital Health technologies and highlight examples of successful applications of these technologies in clinical care. Subsequent chapters build on this foundational understanding by exploring in greater detail their benefits, limitations, and future implications.

ELECTRONIC HEALTH RECORDS

Electronic health record (EHR) systems are digital representations of a patient's medical history maintained by healthcare providers over a defined period. In high-income countries such as the United States (US) and Canada,

 DOI: 10.1201/9781003610519-2

EHRs have been implemented in nearly all care facilities, and the integration of novel features such as artificial intelligence and patient portals are currently under consideration or are being trialed. In other parts of the world, EHRs have seen a more variable uptake because of challenges such as high upfront monetary costs and insufficient accompanying technological and regulatory infrastructure.[1]

An EHR encompasses essential administrative and clinical data relevant to the care provided to the patient, including demographic information, progress notes, diagnostic problems, medications, vital signs, medical history, immunisation records, laboratory results, radiology reports, and even genetics data. In practice, EHRs serve many functions, from mundane administrative tasks such as scheduling patient appointments to supporting advanced patient care through the integration of clinical decision support systems.[2]

In addition to their primary use for day-to-day clinical work, EHRs have also demonstrated value at the organisational and national levels. In terms of standard operations management, EHRs enable the collection of data used to evaluate performance against key metrics, inform research and service improvement priorities, and justify financial and strategic decisions. Along with other sources of data, such as public health data, EHRs provide an important input for big data analytics that can inform priorities in care and research. Recent experiences from the COVID-19 pandemic have also demonstrated the value of EHRs under unprecedented circumstances by enabling more timely and effective communicable disease surveillance.[3]

However, despite the opportunities made possible by the growing availability and routine use of EHRs, notable shortcomings remain that accompany their use. Challenges include heterogeneity in implementation, widespread concerns about data privacy and security, a lack of data standardisation, poor system interoperability, insufficient resources to introduce or maintain the technology involved, and the non-uniformity of training of healthcare workers on both how to use them and best practices. In many settings, even when successful EHR implementation has been achieved, factors such as government regulations, changing incentive schemes, and the added administrative burden on healthcare workers can all influence the value of EHRs over time.[4]

Although EHR uptake and use in geographic and clinical settings will continue to vary, reducing administrative burdens, integrating with novel health devices and patient portals, facilitating more seamless coordination across disparate health services and providers, and improving patient experiences when accessing their medical information are likely to remain key priorities in the future.

TELEHEALTH
Virtual Consultations

Virtual care consultations are defined as Primary Care consultations that occur remotely and are primarily intended to facilitate remote interactions between healthcare providers and patients through digital platforms, such as online conferencing software or telephone calls. Virtual care consultations in Primary Care predate the COVID-19 pandemic, but their use markedly increased in 2020 in response to COVID-19 infection control measures.[5]

Post-pandemic, virtual care consultations have become integral to Primary Care as a mechanism to improve continuity of care, accessibility, and efficiency. In many health systems, they offer an attractive alternative to in-person consultations. For example, virtual care consultations may provide continuity of care for rural populations in the US who might otherwise lack reliable access to primary healthcare.

However, it is crucial to acknowledge that virtual care consultations are no panacea and do come with notable limitations to their use. Certain populations, such as those without reliable internet access or those with poor digital literacy or language barriers, may face disproportionate challenges when utilising virtual care consultations compared with traditional, in-person care.[6]

In recent years, advancements in technology have significantly enhanced virtual consultations' functionality, reliability, and integration into healthcare systems.[7] Emerging telemedicine platforms offer improved interfaces for both patients and providers. The integration of virtual care consultations into existing EHRs has streamlined workflows, enabled improved documentation, and enhanced continuity of care. Digital diagnostic tools, such as remote monitoring devices, have likewise emerged to complement the boom in virtual care consultations.

In light of the increasing emergence of virtual care consultations, medical students and early career clinicians should be equipped with the skills and knowledge to deliver effective care through these consultations. For example, students should consider the differences in establishing rapport and patient-centred communication in virtual versus in-person consultations. Clinicians must familiarise themselves with common virtual examination techniques, recognise their limitations, and adapt their clinical judgement accordingly. The nature of remote consultations can also lead to increased diagnostic uncertainty, particularly in cases where physical examinations or advanced diagnostics are required but unavailable. To address this uncertainty, clinicians should plan to implement robust safety-netting strategies alongside virtual consultation implementation. For example, clear guidance on follow-up steps, escalation plans, and the use of additional diagnostic tools can mitigate the potential risks associated with virtual consultations.

Remote Monitoring

Remote monitoring technologies constitute another type of telehealth that enables clinicians to collect health data from patients at a distance and monitor patient conditions outside of in-person healthcare visits. Wearable devices (e.g., smart watches), sensors (e.g., glucometers), and mobile applications (e.g., medication trackers) have emerged as common remote monitoring technologies. These technologies often automatically collect physiological parameters, such as heart rate and oxygen saturation. This information can then be transferred to healthcare providers for review and intervention if required.

Historically, remote monitoring technologies have largely been applied to monitor individuals with chronic diseases to minimise the patient burden of care and maximise the quality of life. In recent years, the use of remote technologies has expanded into areas such as preventive medicine (e.g., sensors for sleep hygiene) and mental health (e.g., well-being mobile applications). Previous research has suggested that remote monitoring technologies may also prevent acute care admissions, though further research is needed to understand the drivers of variation by disease.[8]

These tools have demonstrated potential to improve healthcare delivery, but several challenges should be recognised. First, data from remote monitoring technologies may not always be accurate. For example, oxygen sensors might inadvertently under-alert healthcare providers to lower-than-normal oxygen saturations for patients with darker skin because of pulse oximeter performance disparities.[9] Second, many forms of remote monitoring rely on the regular use of the device. Certain populations, such as those with dementia or depression, may be more at risk for lower remote monitoring adherence. Finally, as with virtual consultations, different populations may be more or less likely to benefit from the use of remote monitoring technologies due to systemic inequities and access challenges. This discussion on the gaps is not intended to be comprehensive. Rather, it is important to consider the potential challenges associated with the use of any new technology, including remote monitoring, so that strategies to overcome these challenges can be developed before implementation.

MOBILE HEALTH APPLICATIONS (mHEALTH)

mHealth can be defined as the use of mobile and wireless digital technologies to improve health. The potential of mHealth applications (apps) to transform healthcare has been increasingly recognised in recent years. mHealth platforms and apps have been developed for all stages of care provision (from prevention to treatment) and with a multitude of functionalities to support patient care. To categorise such functionalities, the following classification has been proposed: (i) support of clinical diagnosis and/or decision-making,

(ii) improvement of clinical outcomes through behaviour change and enhancement of patient adherence and compliance, (iii) standalone digital therapeutics, and (iv) delivery of disease-related education.[10]

The advantages and limitations of mHealth apps are contingent on their intended purposes. One of their most significant advantages is the possibility of monitoring and managing chronic diseases between healthcare visits.[11] For example, digital diaries enable patients to consistently track their symptoms, which enhances self-awareness about their condition and delivers more precise information to physicians. mHealth apps can serve as a platform to deliver personalised interventions to patients and incorporate strategies, such as gamification and coaching, that can enhance the effectiveness of traditional interventions.

Although mHealth care can provide additional support for patients and healthcare teams, particularly between healthcare visits, this benefit may be inequitably distributed. Even within the same country, lower smartphone ownership among older adults, for example, potentially limits the implementation of mHealth-based interventions.[12]

Despite the existence of several apps developed with the aim of improving health outcomes, only a minority have been developed by experts and adequately evaluated. Although countries such as Germany have implemented systems to allow the prescription of approved apps for medical purposes,[13] in many countries, individual healthcare professionals recommend the use of these apps without formal guidance. Healthcare professionals who intend to recommend mHealth apps in clinical practice should consider factors such as whether the claims of the apps are supported by high-quality scientific evidence, whether the entities developing the app are credible and the development process has been transparent, and whether there is minimal risk to patients and their data.

ARTIFICIAL INTELLIGENCE

Artificial intelligence (AI) refers to the development and application of software algorithms to simulate human cognitive abilities and facilitate complex problem-solving, decision-making, and learning from experience.

AI is not a singular, homogenous technology—rather, it comprises a variety of technical approaches that may be used independently or in conjunction with one another to enable AI to fulfil its intended functions. These approaches have progressed from rudimentary rule-based scripts to more sophisticated techniques such as machine learning, deep learning, and natural language processing.

Machine learning (ML) refers to the ability of computers to 'learn' how to make decisions without the need to be pre-programmed or scripted, imitating how humans would act to accomplish certain tasks. ML can be further categorised into various subtypes depending on the 'learning process' involved (e.g., supervised, unsupervised, or reinforcement).

Neural networks are a more complex form of ML in which problems are solved through a combination of inputs, outputs, variables, and weightings. When multiple neural networks are used together, this is referred to as 'deep learning'.

Deep learning is a subfield of ML that utilises multiple layers of neural networks to allow for the modelling and analysis of complex hierarchical patterns and relationships within datasets. Each layer consists of interconnected nodes that receive data and process it before passing it to the next layer. Deep learning is especially useful in managing problems that require large datasets and pattern recognition that are too complex for conventional ML methods to perform efficiently. Common applications of deep learning currently include image classification, object recognition, and natural language processing.

A clinical concept analogous to deep learning might include a multidisciplinary review of a complex patient. The 'input' is the patient information. The 'output' is the diagnosis based on evaluations weighted in different ways. Instead of one doctor providing their opinion in isolation, the full team weighs in based on their clinical expertise, thereby providing a more well-informed output.

Natural language processing (NLP) is a subfield of AI that enables computers to better interpret, understand, and synthesise human language. NLP draws upon concepts from computer science and linguistics, in combination with ML, to complete a diverse range of tasks that resemble human text and speech. These tasks may range from text generation and translation to speech recognition and content summarisation.

Large Language Models (LLM) and Generative AI

LLM is a particular subset of AI models within the field of NLP intended to support the understanding and generation of human language. LLMs are instrumental to the field of generative AI, a type of AI that can generate content, including text, speech, image, or video. LLMs can interpret, understand, and generate human-like text. In the realm of healthcare, the application of LLMs and generative AI is currently used mostly for aggregating and summarising large amounts of knowledge to inform healthcare providers.

However, despite the many advances in LLMs, some technical shortcomings remain—most concerning of which is the phenomenon of 'hallucinations'. Hallucinations refer to the generation of outputs from AI that are incorrect or a misrepresentation of facts. This is often caused by inadequate training of the AI models, flawed or biased data used in the training, or fundamentally incorrect assumptions incorporated within the model itself.

A clinical concept analogous to LLM might include an incredibly driven medical assistant who is up to date on the recent literature related to your specialty. This assistant not only understands the facts but also can learn patterns and recognise common scenarios. You would certainly want to fact check them because they are not perfect, but their input is still incredibly valuable to manage large volumes of information.

Role of AI in Healthcare

The first application of primitive computer-aids in healthcare settings by physicians can be traced back to the 1960s, but it is in recent years that AI has begun to demonstrate its transformative potential in healthcare. Currently, innovations made possible with AI range from predictive medicine and smart clinical decision-making tools to more efficient healthcare administration and management and advancements in research that utilise big data. Much of these innovations have been made possible through the exponential increase in computation power available, greater connectivity, and the marked growth of patient and personal data resulting from the ubiquity of Digital Health technologies such as EHRs and mobile health devices.

AI has facilitated the handling, analysis, and manipulation of large quantities of patient healthcare data. In practice, this has translated into hastening medical research, allowing more effective monitoring and evaluation of healthcare services, and enabling healthcare providers and policymakers to draw greater insight from troves of data from varying sources once deemed impractical to analyse at scale. In Public Health, the introduction of AI has improved epidemic surveillance by increasing the analytical capacity with which to process the data to identify patterns and predict disease transmission in at-risk populations.

AI advancements have had direct applications in clinical care. For example, deep learning has already demonstrated great promise in the realms of radiology and pathology where image analysis has enabled the automated classification of routine images to support diagnoses (e.g., chest x-rays for pneumonia) and the early detection of possible malignancies.

NLP, in the form of ambient AI, has been used to summarise clinical encounters as an innovative means to meaningfully lessen the administrative workloads of providers.[14] Conversational AI also has the potential to support inbox management for clinicians, such as by prioritising patient messages or generating draft responses.[15] AI has allowed clinicians to act more proactively to prevent the onset of disease, offer treatment for time-sensitive presentations (e.g., stroke), and tailor interventions to better suit the needs of patients based on personal risk profiles and behavioural patterns (i.e., precision medicine).

Despite these promising uses of AI in healthcare, notable hurdles remain that greatly limit its use. Although current levels of AI demonstrate enormous potential in streamlining repetitive tasks and processing vast quantities of data to derive insight for clinicians, AI is still not at the level of sophistication to interpret complex, realistic clinical situations and perform independent decision-making. As AI is inherently dependent on the data that it is provided, managing ethical issues concerning the equity and representativeness of the data on which AI models are trained is essential in ensuring that AI in healthcare benefits all members of society.[16] In addition to these substantial technical issues, gaining regulatory approval, training the healthcare workforce on best practices, integrating AI into existing EHR systems and clinical workflows, and protecting privacy are profound challenges that the technology still needs to overcome.

AI is unlikely to replace clinicians, at least for the foreseeable future. Rather, as AI's presence in healthcare settings continues to grow, akin to the Digital Health technologies that preceded it such as EHRs, it will play a supportive role—namely, augmenting clinicians in their clinical decision-making and management, streamlining workflows to improve work efficiency, and providing innovations to enhance patient experience. AI's role in healthcare is just in its infancy and is likely to evolve rapidly and transform healthcare delivery. The use of AI in healthcare must be carefully governed in collaboration with multidisciplinary stakeholders, including patients, to protect against its associated risks.

CASE STUDY 1 mHEALTH

Supporting Respiratory Allergic Disease Management

Challenge: Patients with respiratory allergic disease (allergic rhinitis or asthma) often rely on self-medication to manage difficult symptoms. Although not fatal, respiratory allergic disease has a significant impact on well-being and can substantially interfere with daily activities.

Solution: MASK-air ('the app') is an mHealth app for patients with respiratory allergic disease that was developed by experts of the Allergic Rhinitis and its Impact on Asthma (ARIA) group.

How It Works:

1. The app includes a daily monitoring questionnaire that assesses the impact of rhinitis and asthma symptoms through validated visual analogue scales (VASs).
2. The app allows users to match their daily medications with country-specific prescribed and over-the-counter medications.

3. If patients opt to link their app data to their electronic health record, then their physician can more easily understand how well-controlled and adherent their patients are between health-care visits.

Impact:

- Augments traditional in-person visits, which is particularly helpful as geopolitical and societal changes increasingly intersect with the provision of healthcare.
- Helps physicians assess whether changes to the treatment plan may be required.
- Can complement and extend many traditional clinical functions such as
  - Supporting clinical diagnosis and decision-making,
  - Monitoring and empowering patient adherence, and
  - Delivering disease-related education.

Conclusion:

MASK-air is one example of how mHealth can contribute to immediate outcomes, such as improved management of chronic diseases[17] and advanced knowledge on patient behaviour related to disease management, while paving the way for longer-term contributions to care, such as using mHealth data to inform future best practices and guidelines.

CASE STUDY 2   APPLICATIONS OF AI IN LOW- AND MIDDLE-INCOME COUNTRIES

Combating Diabetic Retinopathy in India with AI-powered Screening

Challenge: India has a high prevalence of diabetes, leading to a significant number of diabetic retinopathy (DR) cases. DR is a leading cause of preventable blindness, but early detection is crucial for effective treatment. Traditional screening methods are often inaccessible or expensive, especially in rural areas with limited ophthalmologists.

Solution: An Indian health tech startup developed an AI-powered DR screening system that uses fundus cameras. This solution aims to improve access to early detection and diagnosis.

How it Works:
1. Healthcare workers use portable, affordable fundus cameras to capture images of the patient's retina.
2. These images are then analysed by AI algorithms trained on vast datasets of retinal images to detect signs of DR.
3. The system provides a risk assessment for DR and highlights areas of concern.
4. The results are available within minutes, enabling faster diagnosis and referral.
5. The AI platform can be used by non-specialist healthcare workers, which increases screening capacity.

Impact:
- Increased accessibility to DR screening in remote areas with limited specialists.
- Faster and more efficient diagnosis, leading to timely treatment.
- Improved accuracy in DR detection, which potentially reduces misdiagnosis.
- Cost-effective solution compared to traditional screening methods.
- Reduced workload for ophthalmologists, allowing them to focus on treatment.

Conclusion:
This case study highlights the transformative impact of AI in primary healthcare and its ability to improve health outcomes for vulnerable populations. These AI-powered solutions are transforming DR screening in India by improving access to care and potentially saving millions from preventable blindness. By integrating these solutions into existing healthcare systems, India can effectively combat the growing burden of DR.

CASE STUDY 3 AI-POWERED SOFTWARE FOR BREAST CANCER DETECTION

Revolutionising Breast Cancer Screening in South Africa

Challenge: South Africa faces high breast cancer mortality rates, particularly in rural areas with limited access to mammography and skilled personnel. Early detection is crucial for successful treatment, yet many South African women lack access to timely and accurate diagnostic services. Traditional methods, such as mammograms, are often expensive and require specialised equipment and trained radiologists, which are often scarce in many provinces. Delayed diagnosis leads to poorer outcomes.

Solution: A South African company developed AI-powered software for breast cancer detection that uses portable handheld ultrasound devices. This solution increases the accessibility and affordability of screening.

How it Works:

1. General Practitioners or nurses can capture breast images using portable handheld ultrasound probes.
2. Images are uploaded to a cloud platform for AI analysis.
3. AI algorithms identify and provide risk scores for suspicious areas in real-time.
4. The software delivers immediate feedback to healthcare workers.

Impact:

- Increased early detection rates through accessible screening in both urban and rural areas.
- Reduced diagnostic delays due to real-time AI analysis.
- Improved diagnostic accuracy with AI.
- Empowering patients with access to information and supportive resources.

Conclusion:

These AI-driven solutions have the potential to significantly improve breast cancer outcomes in South Africa. By empowering healthcare providers with advanced AI tools, these AI-powered solutions can improve patient outcomes, reduce healthcare costs, and enhance the overall quality of care.

CASE STUDY 4 NOVEL USES OF BIG DATA IN EHRs

Improving Lung Cancer Screening

Challenge: Lung cancer screening using low-dose computed tomography (LDCT) has been shown to reduce mortality rates among smokers. The United States Preventive Services Task Force (USPSTF) recommends LDCT screening for adults aged 50 to 80 years with a 20-pack-year smoking history, including those who quit within the last 15 years. However, broader adoption faces three main challenges: limited radiology capacity, false positives, and overdiagnosis.

Solution: Leumit Health Services, one of the four Health Maintenance Organisations (HMO) in Israel, has developed a predictive model for lung cancer that utilises 20 years of patient data from over one million individuals in its electronic health records.

How it Works: This model, which is trained on historical data from patients diagnosed with lung cancer within two-and-a-half years of a medical visit, incorporates laboratory tests, physical measures, demographic information, medication purchase patterns, lifestyle factors (including smoking), and service utilisation. This comprehensive approach aims to improve the accuracy and efficiency of lung cancer screening and could potentially address the limitations of current standards and enable broader implementation.

The model uses innovative technology to standardise the time trajectory of time-dependent variables. It is based on thousands of variables extracted from patients' electronic records, with key features including patient birth dates, zip codes, smoking status, socioeconomic score, encoded first and last names, the names of their fathers (which provide insights into ethnicity), the frequency of upper respiratory infections, and specific medications purchased, particularly those affecting the respiratory and nervous systems.

Impact: The model claims to identify the top 1% of high-risk individuals with a positive predictive value (PPV) of 3.87% for lung cancer diagnosis within four years, indicating a 12-fold increased risk compared to peers.

Conclusion: Using this model to target high-risk patients may aid in mitigating service shortages, reducing false positives, and improving overall screening effectiveness. This case study highlights the potential of leveraging historical patient data found in EHRs to better inform the use of limited healthcare resources and potentially improve health outcomes.

KEY MESSAGES

- Digital Health technologies have become commonplace in many clinical environments, with electronic health records and clinical decision support tools being routinely used in most high-income countries.

- Digital Health technologies are being introduced in both high-income countries (HIC) and low- and middle-income countries (LMICs) in innovative ways to provide high-quality Primary Care despite resource limitations.
- Technologies such as virtual consultations, which were once used only in select circumstances for specific applications, have seen a steadily increasing uptake post-pandemic in Primary Care.
- Recent innovations such as artificial intelligence, whilst not replacing healthcare workers, are set to alter the role that digital technology plays in healthcare. Health systems must adapt, and healthcare workers must be trained to best use these new tools.

REFERENCES

1. Kerr G, Kulshreshtha N, Greenfield G, et al. Features and frequency of use of electronic health records in Primary Care across 20 countries: a cross-sectional study. *Public Health*. 2024;233:45–53. https://doi.org/10.1016/J.PUHE.2024.05.001.
2. Kwan JL, Lo L, Ferguson J, et al. Computerised clinical decision support systems and absolute improvements in care: meta-analysis of controlled clinical trials. *BMJ*. 2020 Sep 17;370.
3. Madhavan S, Bastarache L, Brown JS, et al. Use of electronic health records to support a public health response to the COVID-19 pandemic in the United States: a perspective from 15 academic medical centers. *J Am Med Inf Assoc*. 2021;28(2):393–401. https://doi.org/10.1093/JAMIA/OCAA287.
4. Kroth PJ, Morioka-Douglas N, Veres S, et al. Association of electronic health record design and use factors with clinician stress and burnout. *JAMA Netw Open*. 2019;2(8):e199609. https://doi.org/10.1001/JAMANETWORKOPEN.2019.9609.
5. Shaver J. The state of telehealth before and after the COVID-19 pandemic. *Primary Care*. 2022;49(4):517. https://doi.org/10.1016/J.POP.2022.04.002.
6. Khoong EC, Butler BA, Mesina O, et al. Patient interest in and barriers to telemedicine video visits in a multilingual urban safety-net system. *J Am Med Inf Assoc*. 2020;28(2):349. https://doi.org/10.1093/JAMIA/OCAA234.
7. Greenhalgh T, Shaw S, Wherton J, et al. Hodkinson I real-world implementation of video outpatient consultations at macro, meso, and micro levels: mixed-method study. *J Med Internet Res*. 2018;20(4):e150.
8. Thomas EE, Taylor ML, Banbury A, et al. Factors influencing the effectiveness of remote patient monitoring interventions: a realist review. *BMJ Open*. 2021;11(8):e051844. https://doi.org/10.1136/BMJOPEN-2021-051844.
9. Holder AL, Wong AKI. The big consequences of small discrepancies: why racial differences in pulse oximetry errors matter. *Crit Care Med*. 2022;50(2):335. https://doi.org/10.1097/CCM.0000000000005447.
10. Rowland SP, Fitzgerald JE, Holme T, et al. What is the clinical value of mHealth for patients? *NPJ Digit Med*. 2020;3(1):1–6. https://doi.org/10.1038/s41746-019-0206-x.
11. Chong SOK, Pedron S, Abdelmalak N, et al. An umbrella review of effectiveness and efficacy trials for app-based health interventions. *NPJ Digit Med*. 2023;6(1):1–11. https://doi.org/10.1038/s41746-023-00981-x.

12. Badr J, Motulsky A, Denis JL. Digital health technologies and inequalities: a scoping review of potential impacts and policy recommendations. *Health Policy.* 2024;146:105122. https://doi.org/10.1016/J.HEALTHPOL.2024.105122; https://doi.org/10.1111/CEA.14135.

13. Schmidt L, Pawlitzki M, Renard BY, et al. The three-year evolution of Germany's digital therapeutics reimbursement program and its path forward. *NPJ Digit Med.* 2024;7(1): 1–8. https://doi.org/10.1038/s41746-024-01137-1.

14. Coiera E, Kocaballi B, Halamka J, et al. The digital scribe. *NPJ Digit Med.* 2018 Oct 16;1(1):58.

15. Sarkar U, Bates DW. Using artificial intelligence to improve Primary Care for patients and clinicians. *JAMA Intern Med.* 2024 Apr 1;184(4):343–4.

16. Panch T, Pearson-Stuttard J, Greaves F, et al. Artificial intelligence: opportunities and risks for public health. *Lancet Digit Health.* 2019;1(1):e13–14. https://doi.org/10.1016/S2589-7500(19)30002-0.

17. Sousa-Pinto B, Jácome C, Pereira AM, et al. Development and validation of an electronic daily control score for asthma (e-DASTHMA): a real-world direct patient data study. *Lancet Digit Health.* 2023;5(4):e227–38. https://doi.org/10.1016/S2589-7500(23)00020-1.

CHAPTER 3

The Role of Digital Health in Patient-Centred Care

Keith Thompson, Hüsna Sarıca Çevik,
Hans Eguia, Bridget L. Ryan,
Moira Stewart, and Tom Freeman

OVERVIEW OF THE PRINCIPLES OF PATIENT-CENTREDNESS IN PRIMARY CARE

Primary Care is characterised by a longitudinal relationship between patients and their family doctors.[1] This relationship goes beyond diagnoses and treatment and involves aspects of medical assessments based on complex human interactions, communication skills, and understanding human behaviours related to illness. The skills, knowledge, and attitudes required for enhancing patient-centred care are outlined in *McWhinney's Textbook of Family Medicine*.[2]

The patient-centred clinical method involves the critical elements of seeing the patient as a whole and understanding their condition, as well as the social, psychological, and personal context of their medical presentation. This requires a longitudinal relationship built upon trust.

The origins of patient-centred medicine arose in response to dissatisfaction with the increasing dominance of a medical approach, emphasising a highly technical pursuit of a diagnosis and often ignoring the patient's needs. The patient-centred clinical method (PCCM) was distinguished from other responses, such as the biopsychosocial model,[3] in that it was not only a model but also a method for delivering patient-centred Primary Care.

The PCCM, as described by Stewart et al.[4] is a guide for clinicians in their work with patients. It presupposes two key mindsets of a clinician: a sharing

DOI: 10.1201/9781003610519-3

of power and a sensitivity to suffering. The PCCM sets out instructions to assist clinicians in providing medical care that encompasses the whole patient in partnership within an ongoing trusting relationship over time. It proposes four components for the clinician to keep in mind: 1) Exploring Health, Disease, and the Illness Experience; 2) Understanding the Whole Person; 3) Finding Common Ground; and 4) Enhancing the Patient-Clinician Relationship (Figure 3.1).

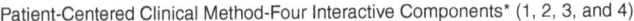

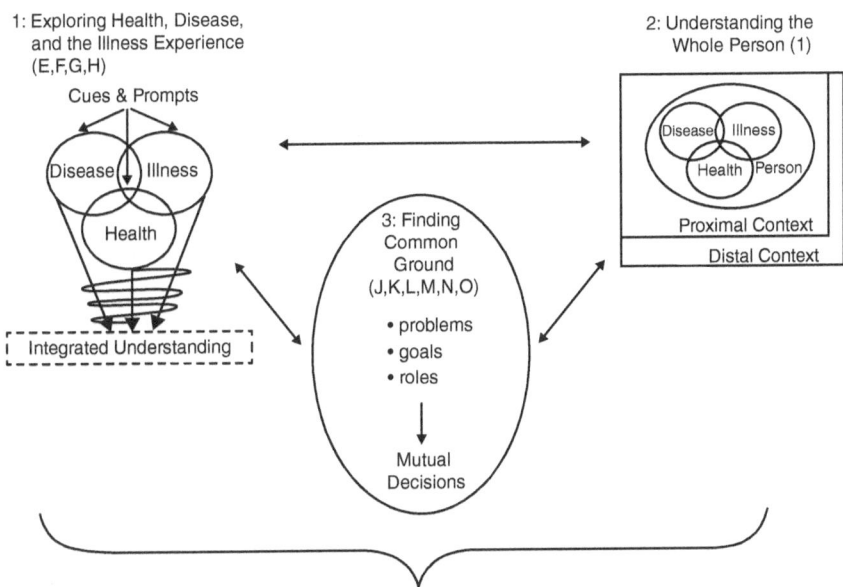

4: Enhancing the Patient-Clinician Relationship

Legend

(A) Telephone care	(1) Health digital literacy
(B) Video care	(J) Point-of-care technologies
(C) Electronic records (EHR and EMR)	(K) AI in imaging
(D) Patient portals	(L) Data science
(E) Wearables	(M) Reminder systems
(F) Blood pressure devices	(N) Digital apps to support lifestyle
(G) Glucometers	(O) Clinical decision support systems.
(H) Cardiac monitors	

FIGURE 3.1 Patient-centred clinical method: the four components. Adapted from Figure 1.1 on page 5 in *Patient-centred Medicine—Transforming the Clinical Method*, Fourth Edition by Stewart M, Brown JB, Weston WW, Freeman TR, Ryan BL, McWilliam CL, McWhinney IR, Copyright (2024) by CRC Press. Reproduced by permission of Taylor & Francis Group.

In this chapter, we make the case that digital technology is both a way of doing things and a method to accomplish a task. The PCCM integrates a humanistic approach with the biomedical approach: it aims to carry out humanistic care while not eschewing evidence-based principles. Digital technologies are often prescriptive, breaking down a process into parts, each carried out by different workers, controlled through management. A patient-centred clinician uses prescriptive technologies, shaping them in the service of humanistic care, recognising how to utilise tools for diagnosis and treatment and when and to what extent to use them.[5]

DIGITAL HEALTH IN PRIMARY CARE AND ITS RELATION TO PATIENT-CENTREDNESS

Technology has always been a part of the relationship between patients and their doctors. Historically, introducing technologies into clinical care was seen as threatening the traditional values of patient-doctor relationships. When new innovations arise, it takes time for them to be "absorbed and integrated into the matrix of craft skills which formed the basis of most technologies".[6]

In his book "In the Hands of Doctors," Paul Stepansky reminds us how the introduction of mercury sphygmomanometers was met with great resistance.[7] Physicians were warned of the potential not only to diagnose a condition that did not really exist based on readings but also to pull physicians away from patients. Stepansky argues, "Physicians who are not patient-centred will assuredly not find themselves pulled toward doctor–patient dialogue through the tools of their specialty. But neither will they become less patient-centred on account of these tools"; "the problem is not in their tools but in themselves".[7]

Digital technologies must align with the core principle of putting patients' needs and preferences at the forefront of clinical interactions by enhancing both access to care and communication between the patient and the care team. These tools should support the personalisation of care and improved efficiency, without compromising efficacy.[8] The adoption and integration of digital technologies into clinical workflows is also determined by the current standard of care and the legal and regulatory policies relevant to the region of practice for the patient encounter.

The COVID-19 pandemic limited face-to-face physical interaction and led to the acceleration of the digital integration of healthcare services, and we see the promise of technology, digital solutions, data science, and artificial intelligence (AI) in personalised, timely, and effective care. AI can help analyse large volumes of patient data to identify trends and patterns and can assist in making accurate diagnoses and personalised treatment recommendations.

With the integration of these digital innovations, it may be possible in the near future to develop unique, personalised plans for patients based on their medical history and socio-behavioural context, leading to improvements in patient outcomes and quality of care.

HOW DIGITAL HEALTH TECHNOLOGIES CAN SUPPORT OR HAMPER PATIENT-CENTRED CARE

Digital Health has changed how patients interact with their healthcare providers and manage their health. With tools like patient portals, mobile apps, and personalised health records, patients can easily access their health information and take a more active role in their own care (patient empowerment). As clinicians, it is important that we know how Digital Health can improve patient engagement and decision-making, leading to better health outcomes and a better quality of life.

Digital Health offers many educational tools to help people better understand their health and make correct clinical decisions.[9] For example, patient portals are websites or apps where patients can access their medical information, letting them check their test results, medication lists, and appointments, and even send messages to their physician. This saves time and helps patients have their own information available without needing extra clinic visits.

Portals have been found to positively influence patients' 1) perceptions of control; 2) comprehension of the care plan; 3) preparation for the visit; 4) adherence to prescriptions; and 5) self-management. The way in which a portal is used by the patient should be mutually agreed upon by patient and clinician to support the patient-clinician relationship.[10]

Personal health records (PHRs) are similar to patient portals but are not limited to a single healthcare institution. PHRs offer patients an overview of their medical history, gathering information, including past diagnoses, treatments, test results, medications, and immunisations, in one secure online platform. For example, Türkiye utilises the digitalised platform e-Nabız, a PHR system that empowers individuals to track their health data for prevention, health promotion, and sharing health records with different physicians.[11]

PHRs are especially useful in the healthcare system when visiting a different doctor; patients can share their medical history, ensuring accurate and timely care. These records help patients make informed decisions by reviewing past diagnoses and treatments.[12] PHRs can allow users to share data with caregivers and contribute to medical research, leveraging their health data to potentially benefit others. Overall, PHRs empower patients to take an active role in their care.[9]

Electronic health records (EHRs) can bring many other advantages to healthcare, such as improving guideline adherence and reducing medication errors.[13] However, there are also negative effects associated with their use: EHRs can decrease rapport and hamper the patient-physician relationship, and physicians complain of increased workload and lower job satisfaction, commonly leading to burnout. Some of the EHR negative effects on the patient-physician relationship may be mitigated by integrating a patient-centred approach while using EHRs.[14]

HOW DIGITAL HEALTH CAN PROMOTE SELF-MANAGEMENT AND PREVENTATIVE CARE

Nowadays, patients can have access to powerful mobile tools that empower them to have a better awareness of their diseases and that can support them with health behaviour change and chronic disease self-management. For example, someone with diabetes can use an app to control their blood sugar levels, get reminders for medications, and see patterns over time in their data. Apps can also help monitor blood pressure, physical activity, or sleep, giving the patient and the physician a clear picture of the patient's condition.

Wearable technologies and AI are key innovations that are accelerating self-management and preventative care. Wearable devices such as smartwatches and biosensors have become everyday tools to help patients and clinicians with "proactive" health management.[15] These devices can monitor vital signs like heart rate, sleep patterns, physical activity, and oxygen levels, helping motivate users to engage in physical activity or remind them to move after sitting too long. Some wireless and wearable devices also enable the use of electrocardiograms by patients to detect cardiac arrhythmias; some allow blood pressure monitoring. An increasingly common device is the continuous blood glucose monitor, that monitors sugar levels in real time, allowing patients to adjust their glycemic control medications. The data collected by these devices can be shared with doctors to make joint decisions to improve health outcomes. In addition, data from wearable technologies and from the patient's medical history can be leveraged by AI to identify patterns and potentially allow health professionals to routinely develop personalised care plans for their patients.

HOW DIGITAL HEALTH CAN EXPAND OR REDUCE ACCESS TO HEALTH CARE SERVICES

Digital Health interventions have the potential to improve the access to and quality of Primary Care services. There are significant differences in Digital Health adoption across countries. Inequalities in internet access, the prevalence of technical problems in systems, the level of digital illiteracy among patients and healthcare providers, and the comprehensiveness of country policies supporting Digital Health play a crucial role in affecting the adoption of Digital Health in primary healthcare service delivery.[16]

During COVID-19, telephone and video consultations in Primary Care increased exponentially. Virtual care has improved access to care for patients with limited mobility and those with lack of transportation or no flexibility to leave work.[17] However, there remains a concern about increasing disparities in access to care for vulnerable patients without telephone or internet coverage, where technology has yet to provide a sufficient answer. Using the PCCM model, it is possible to increase patient-centredness in virtual visits.[18, 19] by lengthening the telephone or video visit and being comfortable with silences (saying "mmm" and nodding); giving attention to psychological issues and concerns; summarising patients' expressions of problems and confirming their understanding of care plans; and taking enough time to attend to patients' emotions during the consultation.

Importantly, Digital Health comes with its own limitations, in what concerns ensuring patients needs are identified, met, and adequate access to care is provided. The following case focuses on the limitations of virtual care, the importance of understanding the context of the patient's condition, and how some features may not be evident using virtual care tools.

CASE STUDY: CAN PATIENT NEEDS BE OVERLOOKED IN VIRTUAL CARE?

A 66-year-old male resides alone at home and has type 2 diabetes, chronic kidney disease, and recently, prostate cancer. The management of diabetes is complicated by challenges with follow-up during COVID-19 and missed appointments often due to work. Virtual visits with the family physician were sometimes over the telephone and other times via video. During phone calls, the patient seemed well and was smiling and amused.

In one recent video call, the patient was in a dimly lit room and seemed to show slight distress with movement but denied significant pain.

Later, the family doctor received a call from the daughter who expressed concerns that her father was not coping well. She described a house in disarray and open sores on his lower leg with edema. She wondered if he could be depressed.

The family physician arranged in-person assessment. On arrival, there was evidence that the patient was struggling with housekeeping tasks. The open areas on his extremity were arterial ulcers, with lower leg edema. The patient agreed to homecare assessments and antibiotics. The daughter described her father's demeanor as improved during the visit but explained how the patient's housekeeping and activities of daily living (ADL) were impaired. The prior virtual visits had failed to disclose the severity of impairment.

This case highlights how an ecosystem of Digital Health tools—virtual visits, gathering data remotely such as BP and glucometer readings, and corresponding with specialists using the EHR—left the clinician distanced from the patient, reducing their ability to see the whole person and understand them in the context of their illness journey. The patient's coping status and the extent of their ADL impairment was evident upon a home visit but was challenging to appreciate using virtual care technology. Digital Health was insufficient to capture the whole story of the patient, which required a humanistic and personal encounter among doctor, patient, and caregivers to adequately address the patient-centred goals.

CONCLUSION

Digital technologies are not incompatible with a patient-centred approach in Primary Care; conversely, they can—and should—work synergistically to improve the quality of care. This chapter subsumed relevant digital technologies into components of the patient-centred clinical method. Digital Health has a key role to play in empowering patients and expanding access to care. The chapter closed with a case study illustrating the importance of hybrid care, highlighting the importance of using virtual approaches to augment rather than replace face-to-face medicine.

KEY MESSAGES

- The patient-centred clinical method is a key component of Primary Care, and technology should enhance this clinical method rather than replace it.
- Digital Health can enhance patient-centred care by empowering patients and improving access to primary healthcare.
- Virtual visits can be conducted in a patient-centred manner by using the patient-centred clinical method.
- Hybrid approaches combining virtual and in-person care are key to identify the elements of patient-centred care that could otherwise be missed in virtual care.

REFERENCES

1. World Health Organization. *Primary health care.* 2022 Aug 11. Cited 2024 Dec 14. Available from: https://www.who.int/news-room/questions-and-answers/item/primary-health-care.

2. McWhinney IR, Freeman T. The patient-centered clinical method. In: McWhinney IR, Freeman T, editors. *McWhinney's textbook of family medicine.* 4th ed. New York: Oxford University Press; 2016. p. 171. https://doi.org/10.1093/med/9780199370689.001.0001.

3. Engel GL. The need for a new medical model: a challenge for biomedicine. *Science.* 1977;196(4286):129–36. https://doi.org/10.1126/science.847460.

4. Stewart M, Brown JB, Weston WW, et al. *Patient-centered medicine: transforming the clinical method.* 4th ed. Boca Raton: CRC Press; 2024.

5. Franklin U. The 1989 CBC Massey lectures: the real world of technology. *CBC Ideas.* Cited 2024 Dec 14. Available from: https://www.cbc.ca/radio/ideas/the-1989-cbc-massey-lectures-the-real-world-of-technology-1.2946845.

6. McWhinney IR. Medical knowledge and the rise of technology. *J Med Philos.* 1978;3(4):294.

7. Helfand DJ. *In the hands of doctors: touch and trust in medical care.* Montclair: Keynote Books, LLC; 2017. ISBN: 978-0-9830807-7-0.

8. McWhinney IR. Primary Care: core values. Core values in a changing world. *BMJ.* 1998 Jun 13;316(7147):1807–9. https://doi.org/10.1136/bmj.316.7147.1807. PMID: 9624075; PMCID: PMC1113320.

9. Hägglund M, McMillan B, Whittaker R, et al. Patient empowerment through online access to health records. *BMJ.* 2022 Sep 29;378:e071531. Cited 2024 Nov 24. Available from: https://www.bmj.com/content/378/bmj-2022-071531.

10. Ryan BL, Brown JB, Terry AL, et al. Implementing and using a patient portal: a qualitative exploration of patient and provider perspectives on engaging patients. *J Innov Health Inform.* 2016 Jul;23(2):534–40.

11. Birinci Ş. A digital opportunity for patients to manage their health: Turkey national personal health record system (The e-Nabız). *Balkan Med J.* 2023 May 8;40(3):215–21. https://doi.org/10.4274/balkanmedj.galenos.2023.2023-2-77. Epub 2023 Apr 28. Erratum in: *Balkan Med J.* 2023 Jul 12;40(4):307. https://doi.org/10.4274/balkanmedj.galenos.2023.0706. PMID: 37114621; PMCID: PMC10175887.

12. Brands MR, Gouw SC, Beestrum M, et al. Patient-centered digital health records and their effects on health outcomes: systematic review. *J Med Internet Res.* 2022 Dec 1;24(12):e43086. Cited 2024 Nov 24. Available from: https://pmc.ncbi.nlm.nih.gov/articles/PMC9816956/.

13. Campanella P, Lovato E, Marone C, et al. The impact of electronic health records on healthcare quality: a systematic review and meta-analysis. *Eur J Public Health.* 2016;26(1):60–4.

14. Duke P, Frankel RM, Reis S. How to integrate the electronic health record and patient-centered communication into the medical visit: a skills-based approach. *Teach Learn Med.* 2013;25(4):358–65.

15. Kang HS, Exworthy M. Wearing the future-wearables to empower users to take greater responsibility for their health and care: scoping review. *JMIR mHealth uHealth.* 2022 Jul 1;10(7):e35684. Cited 2024 Nov 30. Available from: https://pmc.ncbi.nlm.nih.gov/articles/PMC9330198/.

16. Erku D, Khatri R, Endalamaw A, et al. Digital health interventions to improve access to and quality of primary health care services: a scoping review. *Int J Environ Res Public Health.* 2023 Sep 28;20(19):6854. https://doi.org/10.3390/ijerph20196854. PMID: 37835125.

17. Ryan BL, Thompson K, Meredith L, et al. Family physician virtual care during COVID-19 in London-Middlesex, Ontario, Canada: a mixed methods exploration. *Ann Fam Med*. 2022 Apr 1;20(Suppl 1):2863. https://doi.org/10.1370/afm.20.s1.2863.
18. Grundland B, Forsey J, Herzog LS, et al. Patient-centred care turns 30: being informed by person and patient experience in virtual care. In: Hilty D, Mishkind MC, Malik TS, et al., editors. *Virtual mental health care for rural and underserved settings*. Cham: Springer; 2022. Chapter 3. Available from: https://doi.org/10.1007/978-3-031-11984-2.
19. Stewart M, Ryan BL, Freeman TR. Patient-centered approaches in the face of new technologies. In: Stewart M, Brown JB, Weston WW, et al., editors. *Patient-centered medicine: transforming the clinical method*. 4th ed. Boca Raton, FL: CRC Press; 2024. Chapter 9. pp. 171–9.

CHAPTER 4

Improving Clinical Effectiveness Through Digital Interventions

Nana Kwame Ayisi-Boateng,
Eric Kojo Nsa Oduro,
Obed Kwabena Offe Amponsah,
Douglas Aninng Opoku, Jacopo Demurtas,
and Benedict Hayhoe

Digital Health tools are transforming healthcare in the way that they support patients and clinicians and improve clinical effectiveness. Some of the technologies with the strongest evidence for improved outcomes include digital self-management support tools for patients with chronic conditions and Clinical Decision Support Systems (CDSS) for clinicians.

DIGITAL SELF-MANAGEMENT SUPPORT TOOLS TO IMPROVE CLINICAL EFFECTIVENESS

Modern medicine requires patients to play a significant role in the management of their healthcare because of the heightened burden of chronic disease on health systems.[1] This includes managing their symptoms, living a healthy lifestyle, and adhering to treatment schedules and medication. Rapid population growth and aging have resulted in increased demand for primary healthcare, putting further burden on health systems. Hence, patients' ability to use digital tools to take a more active role in the optimisation of their clinical outcomes may help to reduce this burden.

DOI: 10.1201/9781003610519-4

With the aid of mHealth tools, people now have access to a variety of digital tools to practice self-management and monitor the progress of their health through different metrics. These Digital Health tools may employ resources like health education or behaviour change techniques to stimulate practices that are beneficial to their chronic disease management, such as medication adherence or physical activity, and can ultimately improve their clinical outcomes.

Digital self-management support tools (DSMSTs) are technologies and/or platforms designed to aid people to achieve better clinical outcomes by supporting them managing their health or general well-being. They may be used by patients with chronic medical conditions to monitor their health status, adopt a healthier lifestyle, and help manage different tasks related to their disease. Evidence indicates that digital self-management tools for patients with chronic diseases can effectively improve risk factor control (e.g., glycemic control in diabetes patients, blood pressure),[2,3] although evidence is weaker in populations with digital barriers.[4]

In instances where patients have access to information about their health, educational resources, and the capacity to self-manage, they may be more likely to participate in their care, adhere to treatment plans, and make the right decisions to improve their general well-being.[5] The use of DSMSTs can help patients monitor their health outside of clinical settings and allow them to monitor vital signs and other health parameters, symptoms, medication adherence, and other metrics.

With DSMSTs, patients can generate data that can be shared with their primary healthcare providers. Data generated from digital self-management tools may be helpful for patients to identify trends and patterns, particularly if analysed with the assistance of their primary healthcare provider. Having access to this health information can be helpful for primary healthcare providers to guide them in making clinical decisions, including diagnosis and timely interventions, and to tailor treatment and management regimens to meet patient needs. In addition, DSMSTs' data may help monitor whether patients are responding to treatment or not, which can aid decisions about optimising treatment plans. DSMSTs can therefore support one of the core tenets of Family Medicine—to provide patient-centred care.[6]

CLINICAL DECISION SUPPORT SYSTEMS FOR CLINICIANS— CAN THEY IMPROVE CLINICAL EFFECTIVENESS?

Clinical decision support systems (CDSS) are typically integrated into electronic health records to assist clinicians by providing real-time guidance. CDSS vary from pop-up alerts about serious drug interactions or allergies to more complex systems that incorporate clinical prediction rules. CDSS can prompt clinicians to deliver evidence-based care and have been shown to be effective at increasing the number of patients receiving desired care (by about 6%) and those achieving guideline-based targets (e.g., blood pressure, lipid control).[7]

CDSS are now also becoming available to healthcare providers on mobile devices at the point of care, particularly in low- and middle-income countries. The use of mobile CDSS by providers can potentially improve adherence to treatment protocols, but the evidence is still growing in this area.[8]

More recent innovations include artificial intelligence (AI)-powered CDSS, with numerous studies indicating good algorithmic performance. However, evidence is still sparse on the effects of AI decision support on patient care, with only a few randomised controlled trials reporting patient-relevant benefits (e.g., in depression treatment and pain management) and trials generally underreporting harms.[9] Despite the growing enthusiasm for the promising role of AI CDSSs in healthcare, more robust trials are needed that show improvements in health outcomes, and more research is needed on the barriers to and facilitators of their successful implementation.

CASE STUDIES

Family Practice Model in Kumasi, Ghana

The University Hospital at the Kwame Nkrumah University of Science and Technology, Kumasi, Ghana has implemented a DSMST through a family practice model (FPM). This 135-bed Primary Care facility, which serves students, staff, and their dependents, faced challenges with continuity of care as patients were seen by different doctors in the Outpatient Department; this led to repeated medical histories, limited patient-doctor relationships, and impaired quality of care.

To address these issues, the hospital implemented an FPM that assigned each family to a specific Family Doctor, with availability for virtual consultations. Additionally, the FPM includes a web app accessible on mobile phones and computers designed to facilitate disease management tasks, including the online scheduling of appointments. In emergencies, the duty doctor updates the family doctor to ensure continuity of care.

Since its implementation, the FPM has reported positive outcomes, including reduced waiting and processing times at the hospital, less stress for patients seeking healthcare, increased client satisfaction, enhanced quality of care, improved doctor–patient relationships, and continuity of care. By investing in health information technology and ongoing provider training, the University Hospital believes to have advanced patient-centred care, supporting the broader goal of universal health coverage in Ghana.

mDiabetes Initiative in Senegal

Another successful case scenario is the mDiabetes Senegal initiative, which is a notable example of a DSMST that has significantly improved health outcomes for people with diabetes in Senegal. Launched in 2014, this programme uses a short message service and voice messages to provide daily recommendations on diabetes management, especially during challenging periods like Ramadan.[10]

The initiative aims to address the high prevalence of diabetes in Senegal, where an estimated 400,000 people are affected, but only a fraction receives proper treatment. By offering personalised advice and reminders, mDiabetes helps patients better manage their condition, leading to improved glycemic control and reduced complications.

The program has been effective in enhancing diabetes management, with participants reporting better adherence to treatment plans and healthier lifestyle choices. The success of mDiabetes highlights the potential of digital tools in supporting chronic disease management in resource-limited settings.[10]

THE NEED FOR EVIDENCE-BASED PRACTICES AND CLINICAL GUIDELINES IN THE DIGITAL ERA

In recent years, there has been advancement in the use and capacity of digital tools that the world has not previously experienced. In healthcare, the widespread use of electronic health records (EHRs), artificial intelligence (AI), telehealth, and large-scale data analysis are some of the notable developments.[11, 12] AI-based diagnostic systems have shown exciting potential in supporting cancer diagnoses and interpreting radiology investigations.[13] However, to ensure that these tools become mainstream and more reliably support patient care, they need to be robustly evaluated and demonstrate patient benefits with minimal harm. This is because although these new tools and innovations have the potential to revolutionise healthcare, they may be misused, provide inconsistent results, or create unintended consequences that are unacceptable in healthcare. In this era, we need strong reliance on evidence-based practices and clinical practice guidelines to ensure that we are measured in our adoption of digital advancements in favor of optimal patient care.

Evidence-based healthcare integrates the training and expertise of healthcare workers with patients' values and preferences and with the best available evidence obtained from the scientific literature.[14] Clinical guidelines, which form an essential part of evidence-based practice, offer information that supports the use of evidence in making clinical decisions. Guidelines provide not only clear direction regarding when to use which intervention for optimal patient care but also the caveats to such directives based on objective evidence.

The rapid advancements of digital technologies, particularly in healthcare, make it essential to develop evidence-based guidelines that can inform clinical practice. Guidelines need to be credible and address both the benefits and harms of the use of digital technologies in healthcare. Biases and conflicts of interest must be carefully handled to facilitate confidence in the final guideline. Comprehensive stakeholder engagement, a robust evidence base, and updates once new evidence becomes available are also essential.

More than ever, evidence-based guidelines are needed to ensure that advancements in technology do not adversely impact the improved patient outcomes for which they are intended. The pace of scientific discovery and technological advancements make it difficult for clinicians to keep up with the most recent literature. Additionally, differences in the interpretation of Digital Health studies may lead to variability in clinical practice among practitioners, potentially affecting the quality of care. Guidelines are essential to support clinicians in the use of digital technologies in their clinical practice and enhance high-quality care delivery.

REFERENCES

1. Taylor SJ, Pinnock H, Epiphaniou E, et al. A rapid synthesis of the evidence on interventions supporting self-management for people with long-term conditions (PRISMS practical systematic review of self-management support for long-term conditions). *Health Serv Deliv Res.* 2014 Dec;2(53):1–580.
2. Siopis G, Moschonis G, Eweka E, et al. Effectiveness, reach, uptake, and feasibility of digital health interventions for adults with hypertension: a systematic review and meta-analysis of randomised controlled trials. *Lancet Digit Health.* 2023 Mar 1;5(3):e144–59.
3. Tarricone R, Petracca F, Svae L, et al. Which behaviour change techniques work best for diabetes self-management mobile apps? Results from a systematic review and meta-analysis of randomised controlled trials. *EBioMed.* 2024 May 1;103.
4. Khoong EC, Olazo K, Rivadeneira NA, et al. Mobile health strategies for blood pressure self-management in urban populations with digital barriers: systematic review and meta-analyses. *NPJ Digit Med.* 2021 Jul 22;4(1):114.
5. Paterick TE, Patel N, Tajik AJ, et al. Improving health outcomes through patient education and partnerships with patients. *Bayl Univ Med Cent Proceed.* 2017 Jan 1;30(1):112–13. Taylor & Francis.
6. Švab I, Cerovečki V. Person-centred care, a core concept of family medicine. *Eur J General Pract.* 2024 Dec 31;30(1):2393860.
7. Kwan JL, Lo L, Ferguson J, et al. Computerised clinical decision support systems and absolute improvements in care: meta-analysis of controlled clinical trials. *BMJ.* 2020 Sep 17;370.

8. Agarwal S, Glenton C, Tamrat T, et al. Decision-support tools via mobile devices to improve quality of care in primary healthcare settings. *Cochrane Database Syst Rev.* 2021;7(7):CD012944.

9. Wilhelm C, Steckelberg A, Rebitschek FG. Benefits and harms associated with the use of AI-related algorithmic decision-making systems by healthcare professionals: a systematic review. *Lancet Reg Health Europe.* 2025 Jan 1;48:101145.

10. WHO Africa. *mDiabetes, an innovative program to improve the health of people with diabetes in Senegal.* Brazzaville: WHO Africa; 2016.

11. Sharma A, Harrington RA, McClellan MB, et al. Using digital health technology to better generate evidence and deliver evidence-based care. *J Am Coll Cardiol.* 2018;71:2680–90.

12. Ho D, Quake SR, McCabe ERB, et al. Enabling technologies for personalized and precision medicine. *Trends Biotechnol.* 2020;38:497–518. Accessed 2024 Dec 17. Available from: http://www.cell.com/article/S0167779919303166/fulltext.

13. Rajpurkar P, Irvin J, Ball RL, et al. Deep learning for chest radiograph diagnosis: a retrospective comparison of the CheXNeXt algorithm to practicing radiologists. *PLoS Med.* 2018;15:e1002686. Accessed 2024 Dec 16. Available from: https://journals.plos.org/plosmedicine/article?id=10.1371/journal.pmed.1002686.

14. Sackett DL, Rosenberg WMC, Gray JAM, et al. Evidence based medicine: what it is and what it isn't. *BMJ Br Med J.* 1996;312:71. Accessed 2024 Dec 16. Available from: https://pmc.ncbi.nlm.nih.gov/articles/PMC2349778/.

CHAPTER 5

Safety and Unintended Consequences

Ulrik Bak Kirk, Rebecca Payne,
Ana Ferreira, Andree Rochfort,
and Nancy Matillya

SAFETY AND SECURITY IN THE DIGITAL ERA

Imagine the scene: Alexander Graham Bell, standing by his groundbreaking invention, spills sulfuric acid on himself and, in a moment of urgency, makes what is by many people considered history's first telemedical consult: "Watson, come here, I want you". This was not just the dawn of the telephone but also the birth of telemedicine, with Bell unknowingly setting in motion a legacy of remote medical assistance.[1]

A few years later, on November 29, 1879, *The Lancet* published a report detailing how a concerned mother used the telephone in a similar way. Fearing her baby might have croup, she enlisted a family member to call a physician, who famously responded, "Lift the child to the telephone and let me hear it cough".[2] By simply listening over the line, the doctor was able to reassure her that it was not croup, making a remote diagnosis and providing peace of mind without stepping into their home.

Fast forward to today, and telemedicine has moved from novelty to necessity. The COVID-19 pandemic drove healthcare to adapt rapidly, moving from face-to-face appointments to an array of remote consultation methods—by phone, video, or digital portals. The transformation has opened new doors for patient access and convenience but has also introduced challenges and risks that healthcare providers must navigate with care. In this chapter, we explore the unintended consequences of this digital shift in Primary Care.

DOI: 10.1201/9781003610519-5

From issues of patient safety to unforeseen risks, we examine embracing the promise of Digital Health without losing sight of its potential pitfalls.

GLOBAL PERSPECTIVES ON UNINTENDED CONSEQUENCES OF DIGITAL HEALTH TECHNOLOGIES

Unintended consequences of Digital Health technologies frequently emerge at the intersection of technological capabilities and healthcare systems.[3] These include errors caused by poorly designed interfaces, data fragmentation, workflow disruptions, inequities in technology adoption, and increased administrative burdens. Addressing these issues is crucial for healthcare providers, policymakers, and educators worldwide.

Alert Fatigue and System Challenges

Digital Health technologies can introduce new patient safety risks due to data entry errors, fragmented displays, and automated alert fatigue (i.e., a situation where people become desensitised to frequent alerts or warnings) in electronic health records (EHRs), leading to medication errors and diagnostic delays.[4] In Australia, adverse events related to health information technology (IT), such as missed drug interactions and decision-support errors, have often been attributed to user interface and system interoperability challenges. Misaligned health system configurations and inadequate software updates further exacerbate these risks.[5]

Unequal Access

While telemedicine has expanded access to care, it has also exposed deep-rooted inequities. A study of the Text4Life program for maternal health in Nigeria revealed that cultural norms and gender biases influence program outcomes, which emphasises the need for inclusive technology design.[6] Similarly, the rapid adoption of telehealth platforms like NHS Scotland's Near Me during the COVID-19 pandemic not only enhanced healthcare access but also highlighted issues such as digital exclusion due to infrastructure and literacy gaps.[7] Vulnerable populations, including many rural residents and the elderly, remain underserved in such contexts.[8]

Increased Staff Workload

Workflow challenges persist with the introduction of digital tools. For example, online consultations often increase administrative workloads instead of reducing them, causing frustration among healthcare providers.[9]

Loss of the Human Element in Healthcare

The increasing reliance on digital healthcare tools has raised concerns about losing the human element in care delivery. The absence of face-to-face interactions can hinder healthcare providers' ability to detect subtle physical, mental, and social symptoms. Delays in addressing health concerns through online systems, coupled with perceptions of impersonal care, may discourage patients from sharing critical health information.[10] Sensitive discussions, such as delivering distressing news, are often better conducted in person.

Challenges for Healthcare Relationships and Systems

Digital consultations can strain provider-patient relationships by limiting personal interactions. Trust and rapport may suffer, especially when family caregivers are excluded from Digital Health processes. Moreover, fragmented systems and insufficient staff training further disrupt care coordination, as evidenced by UK general practice settings where digital tools have created additional administrative burdens and complicated patient management.[11]

What Educators and Curriculum Designers Can Do

To minimise these unintended consequences, medical educators should integrate Digital Health topics into healthcare curricula. This includes data privacy, digital communication, and maintaining patient-centred care in a digital environment. Training programs should emphasise system design principles that support both healthcare teams and patients to ensure that Digital Health's potential is realised while minimising associated risks.[12]

CLINICAL CARE QUALITY AND RISK ASSESSMENT

As Digital Health technologies reshape the clinical landscape, they bring both opportunities and challenges for maintaining and enhancing care quality. Quality of care incorporates safety, timeliness, effectiveness, the efficient use of available resources, equity, person-centred care, and sustainable healthcare practices. Quality improvement and clinical risk management are key aspects of a physician's practice.

Table 5.1 provides an overview of the concepts and issues regarding safety and the unintended consequences of teleconsultation, including a non-exhaustive list of actions that can be taken to manage the associated clinical risks.[13,14]

TABLE 5.1 Overview of the Safety Issues and Mitigation Actions in Teleconsultation

Item	Issue	Action
Medical malpractice insurance	Medico-legal indemnity	Check you are covered
Guidance and standards, ethics, regulation, business models, professionalism	Competence, quality, safety, regulation, ethics, rapport, inexperience, uncertainty	Ensure compliance with current local regulatory and ethical requirements, privacy, confidentiality, continuity, coordination of care, scope of care
	Electronic/online prescribing	Data protection
	Interoperability between systems and multidisciplinary team	Feedback and complaint process, disclosure and follow-up of incidents and adverse events, quality improvement
	Patient sees professionalism in clinical setting	Safe documentation
		Safe electronic prescribing
		Education and training (including safe clinical assessment, clinical examinations, patient self-testing, home equipment)
		Research that includes patient perspectives
Preparedness before beginning the teleconsultation	Introductions	Physician gives patient their name and registration status
	Ensure correct patient and readiness/ acceptability	Consent
	The patient may not appreciate that the virtual/ teleconsultation is a real consultation	Physician informs the patient that this is a clinical consultation and acknowledges possible limitations
	Shared decision-making	Additional actions if indicated, such as tests and physical examinations, are agreed and arranged during the consultation as would normally happen in a face-to-face consultation
	Know which scenarios are inappropriate for teleconsultation	Know when to decline a teleconsultation and convert it to an in-person consultation

Specific clinical scenarios such as language barriers, literacy and cognitive disability, urgent care, first consultation with a new/unknown patient, some people with complex multiple morbidities, other patient groups	Identify clinical risk	Adapt the provision of digital healthcare for the needs of your practice's populations, e.g., rural isolated, urban deprived, etc. Utilise validated assessment tools with patients Know when to decline a teleconsultation and convert it to an in-person encounter
Physician preparedness	Workload burden Adequate staffing and resources Wellbeing and mindset Technology and equipment	Workload management Time management Resources for connectivity Training and updates Avoid physician fatigue

CASE STUDY   COMMUNICATION, LITERACY, AND LANGUAGE

Jane is a 47-year-old woman who has a mild learning disability and has lived alone since the death of her mother. When she needs to see a doctor, she has previously appeared at the surgery where the staff know her and have always slotted her in when needed. One morning, Jane develops an itchy rash. She arrives at the surgery and is told that the doctor will telephone her later. She receives a phone call later that morning. Jane struggles to describe her rash to the doctor and becomes flustered when questioned, answering "yes" to everything she is asked. The doctor asks Jane to send her a photo, but although Jane can use the camera on her phone, she does not understand how to send the photo to the link supplied by the doctor. Because Jane has previously had eczema, the doctor decides that it is probably a recurrence and supplies steroid and emollient creams. Jane actually has scabies, and the rash becomes worse with the treatment. Eventually, Jane attends the hospital's emergency department where the correct diagnosis is made.

Good communication is vital for good general practice. Remote technologies can make this more challenging, particularly where there are existing impediments to communication such as language non-concordance between clinician and patient, patients at the extremes of age, and where communication is impaired by a disability such as learning disabilities, autism, or deafness.[15] Even patients who usually communicate well by phone, video, or text-based messaging can struggle when in pain or unwell. When communication is facilitated through a third party such as a carer or relative, important details can be missed or misrepresented. These challenges can result in the clinician not getting the full clinical picture, leading to misdiagnosis, or an incorrect assessment of the acuity of a disease. Before ending a call, the clinician should ask themself: "Do I have all the information I need? Do I need to see this patient in-person?"

Safety in remote consulting can be considered at the level of the patient, the clinician, and the wider system:

1. **Patient**: When a patient has an unstable chronic disease, complex co-morbidities, or communication challenges because of age (the very young and the elderly), language non-concordance with the clinician, learning difficulties, or illness, gaining a clear picture during a remote consultation is challenging. Adding in video can sometimes be helpful, but the clinician should ask themself whether they have enough information to safely treat the patient. If not, then they will need an additional in-person

assessment. Multiple remote consultations for the same problem should be avoided—a good rule is "Three strikes and you're in"—i.e., no more than three remote consultations for the same problem without an in-person assessment. Certain diseases are particularly risky when managed remotely, for example, chest pain, breathing difficulties, abdominal pain, a new psychosis, and the long-term management of diabetes. Remote care can have benefits in palliative care provision but should supplement rather than replace in-person consultations.

2. **Clinician**: Remote care introduces new challenges for the clinician. To practice safely, the clinician will need excellent communication skills honed for the remote medium that they have adopted; for example, video and telephone consultations require different ways of communicating attention and listening. Interruptions must be minimised, and the temptation to multitask should be avoided. When a diagnosis has been made remotely, it is wise to treat it as provisional until confirmed in person. Particular risks include failing to recognise both urgency and clinical findings in remote consultations. There is also a risk of over/under prescribing and over/under investigating. In circumstances where clinical resources are limited, for example, no in-person consultations available that day, clinicians are at particular risk of inappropriately managing patients remotely.

3. **System**: Safe remote care happens within systems designed and optimised to offer care in this way. Adequate infrastructure such as sufficient telephone lines, headsets, and dual screens is required. Processes need to be adapted for remote care delivery; for example, when a patient might be handed a prescription or referral in-person, consideration must be given as to how to replicate this process in the virtual world. Staff need adequate training, and consideration must be given to vulnerable patients and how they can access care.

TECHNOLOGY: FROM A DETERRENT TO A PROMOTER OF TELEMEDICINE

Table 5.2 highlights the dual role of technology in telemedicine as both an enabler of flexible, accessible, and innovative care and a source of significant challenges. These challenges centre around privacy concerns and the main cybersecurity dimensions of *confidentiality, integrity, availability,* and *trust.*

Technologies can promote efficiency and trust in telemedicine as they allow flexibility of choice, comfort, and privacy, and they increase the potential for compliance with current regulatory requirements in real clinical settings.

TABLE 5.2 Technology and Telemedicine: Challenges and Opportunities

Aspects	Challenges	Opportunities to consider
Privacy & Confidentiality	Lack of private physical spaces to discuss sensitive matters (e.g., children, mental health, etc.) Fear of privacy/cybersecurity breaches The need to get undressed in front of a camera for physical examination The use of different devices (smartphones, laptops, tablets), which introduces their own vulnerabilities that interfere with video communication or that store sensitive data in non-protected spaces Context and technical infrastructure can integrate other vulnerabilities (e.g., unsecured Wi-Fi at an airport)	Patients can seek care anonymously Patients can be more comfortable and talk more freely in the privacy of their homes Patients can control the level of exchange they prefer, by turning the video on or off *Measures*: authentication; access control; encryption; virtual private networks (VPNs); privacy enhancing technologies (PET) and monitoring
Authenticity & Integrity	Hard to confirm participants' identity (camera off, images/profiles can be tampered with) Lack of adequate technical resources for video communication Finding/sharing data may be difficult as they can be spread over different physical and virtual spaces, in different formats Lack of accurate/complete data can negatively impact diagnosis or therapeutic outcomes	With video and sound, identity can confirmed Patients may have access to various records at the moment of consultation and share them at that time *Measures*: authentication; access control; digital signatures; VPNs; input validation; secure storage and monitoring
Availability	Technology is fallible, and hardware and software errors/failures are prone to happen Ransomware attacks often block access to clinical settings and infrastructures Uninvited users disrupt meetings If medical records are not accessible to authorised professionals, then health procedures may be delayed	With technology, telemedicine can happen anywhere at any time Patients' records can be stored in distributed secure databases for easier access *Measures*: strong backup policies/mechanisms; redundant equipment; personalised access control and monitoring
Trust	Challenges can negatively impact trust	Opportunities can positively impact trust

Investment in state-of-the-art technology is also necessary. Most importantly, individuals' literacy and awareness are required regarding best practices for privacy protection and cyberattack prevention.

MITIGATION STRATEGIES AND FORWARD-LOOKING APPROACHES

To harness the benefits of Digital Health technologies while minimising risks, healthcare systems must adopt proactive measures:

- **Guidelines:** Local health systems and services need to develop guidance for clinicians, administrators, and others involved in the provision of digital healthcare.
- **Tools:** Clinically validated tools need to be available for the remote assessment of patients, similarly to how the Centor criteria are used in face-to-face care to identify the likelihood of a bacterial infection in patients complaining of a sore throat.
- **Design Principles:** User-centred design and robust usability testing are essential to prevent errors and optimise workflows.
- **Training and Education:** Equipping providers with digital literacy skills and fostering a culture of safety can mitigate resistance and enhance adoption.
- **Policy and Regulation:** Frameworks that emphasise safety, equity, and patient-centredness can guide technology deployment while addressing disparities.
- **Monitoring and Feedback:** Continuous evaluation and feedback loops enable systems to adapt to emerging challenges.

KEY MESSAGES

- Keep in mind that communication and clinical assessment can be more challenging in remote settings. Be mindful of the limitations when delivering care remotely.
- Digital technologies not only offer opportunities but also introduce new safety concerns. Proactively identifying these challenges allows for mitigating them, thereby enhancing the safety of care delivery.
- Medical educators should integrate Digital Health topics into curricula, with a focus on data privacy, digital communication, and patient-centred care to harness the benefits while minimising the potential risks.
- Incorporating patient perspectives into medical education, training, research, and clinical risk assessment for digital con-

sultations is essential to ensure patient-centred care that is both geographically and culturally sensitive.

- Investment and resources are necessary to improve digital literacy, protect privacy, and prevent security breaches in telemedicine. Other key factors for seamless efficient telemedicine include better access to state-of-the-art technology for patients and physicians.

NOTE: ChatGPT was used for language editing purposes.

REFERENCES

1. Dorman T. Telemedicine. *Anesthesiol Clin N Am*. 2020 Sept 1;18(3):663–76. https://doi.org/10.1016/S0889-8537(05)70185-1.
2. *The Lancet*. 1879 Nov 29;114(2935):787–822.
3. Ziebland S, Hyde E, Powell J. Power, paradox and pessimism: on the unintended consequences of digital health technologies in   Primary Care. *Soc Sci Med*. 2021 Nov;289:114419. https://doi.org/10.1016/j.socscimed.2021.114419. Epub 2021 Sep 23. PMID: 34619631.
4. Leighton C, Cooper A, Porter A, et al. Effectiveness and safety of asynchronous telemedicine consultations in general practice: a systematic review. *BJGP Open*. 2024 Apr 25;8(1). https://doi.org/10.3399/BJGPO.2023.0177. PMID: 37783479; PMCID: PMC11169987.
5. Kim MO, Coiera E, Magrabi F. Problems with health information technology and their effects on care delivery and patient outcomes: a systematic review. *J Am Med Inform Assoc*. 2017 Mar 1;24(2):246–50. https://doi.org/10.1093/jamia/ocw154. PMID: 28011595; PMCID: PMC7651955.
6. Udenigwe O, Okonofua FE, Ntoimo LFC, et al. Understanding gender dynamics in mHealth interventions can enhance the sustainability of benefits of digital technology for maternal healthcare in rural Nigeria. *Front Glob Womens Health*. 2022 Sep 6;3:1002970. https://doi.org/10.3389/fgwh.2022.1002970. PMID: 36147776; PMCID: PMC9485539.
7. Fang ML, Walker M, Wong KLY, et al. Future of digital health and community care: exploring intended positive impacts and unintended negative consequences of COVID-19. *Healthc Manage Forum*. 2022 Sep;35(5):279–85. https://doi.org/10.1177/08404704221107362. Epub 2022 Jul 1. PMID: 35775162; PMCID: PMC9253718.
8. Huibers L, Bech BH, Kirk UB, et al. Contacts in general practice during the COVID-19 pandemic: a register-based study. *Br J Gen Pract*. 2022 Oct 27;72(724):e799–808. https://doi.org/10.3399/BJGP.2021.0703. PMID: 36253113; PMCID: PMC9591020.
9. Turner A, Morris R, Rakhra D, et al. Unintended consequences of online consultations: a qualitative study in UK Primary Care. *Br J Gen Pract*. 2022 Jan 27;72(715):e128–37. https://doi.org/10.3399/BJGP.2021.0426. PMID: 34903520; PMCID: PMC8813120.
10. Abdelaziz S, Garfield S, Neves AL, et al. What are the unintended patient safety consequences of healthcare technologies? A qualitative study among patients, carers and healthcare providers. *BMJ Open*. 2024 Nov 27;14(11):e089026. https://doi.org/10.1136/bmjopen-2024-089026. PMID: 39608995; PMCID: PMC11603710.

11. Payne R, Dakin F, MacIver E, et al. Challenges to quality in contemporary, hybrid general practice: a multi-site longitudinal case study. *Br J Gen Pract*. 2024 Nov 18. https://doi.org/10.3399/BJGP.2024.0184. Epub ahead of print. PMID: 39117426; PMCID: PMC11583039.

12. Kirk UB, Payne R, Tweedie JA, et al. 'A tool for every job': use of video in urgent Primary Care. *Br J Gen Pract*. 2024 Sep 26;74(747):443–4. https://doi.org/10.3399/bjgp24X739473. PMID: 39327075; PMCID: PMC11441613.

13. Cascella LM. *Bridging the digital divide: creating a personalized telehealth experience*. MedPro Group. Accessed 2024 Dec 19. Available from: https://www.medpro.com/bridging-digital-divide-telehealth.

14. Telemedicine. *Phone and video consultations: a guide for doctors*. Irish Medical Council 2020. Accessed 2024 Dec 19. Available from: https://www.medicalcouncil.ie/news-and-publications/publications/overview/telemedicine-for-doctors-booklet.pdf.

15. Payne R, Clarke A, Swann N, et al. Patient safety in remote Primary Care encounters: multimethod qualitative study combining safety I and safety II analysis. *BMJ Qual Saf*. 2024 Aug 16;33(9):573–86. https://doi.org/10.1136/bmjqs-2023-016674. PMID: 38050161; PMCID: PMC11347200.

CHAPTER 6

Equity and the Digital Divide

Steven van de Vijver, Paulien Tensen,
Raquel Gómez Bravo, Francisca Gaifém,
Pratyush Kumar, and Mercy Wanjala

EXPLORING DIGITAL HEALTH EQUITY

The World Health Organization advocates the use of Digital Health technologies (DHTs) for advancing population health, but concerns about inequitable outcomes persist. Differences in access and use of DHTs across different demographic groups, if not addressed, will lead to a worsening of already existing health inequities. This chapter explores the key definitions, frameworks, and dimensions of Digital Health equity to establish a foundational understanding for evaluating access, usability, and outcomes, with a focus on marginalised and vulnerable populations.

Digital Health equity can be defined as an equal opportunity for individuals to benefit from the knowledge and practices related to the development and use of DHTs to improve health. It is imperative to identify and address the disparities that result from unequal access to devices, internet connectivity, and digital literacy.

If equity considerations are not explicitly integrated into the design, implementation, and evaluation of DHTs, then the rapid proliferation of these technologies risks exacerbating rather than mitigating existing health disparities, especially for vulnerable groups. Examples of key vulnerable groups include racial/ethnic minorities, socioeconomically disadvantaged populations, underserved rural populations, sexual and gender minorities, older people, migrants and refugees, mental health service users, frequent users of health

 DOI: 10.1201/9781003610519-6

services, and the unemployed. Factors that exacerbate inequities among these vulnerable populations include health access (and barriers), algorithmic bias, digital and general health literacy, and security, surveillance and safety.

Frameworks for Understanding and Evaluating Digital Health Equity

Several frameworks have been proposed to conceptualise and evaluate Digital Health equity. The Digital Health Equity Framework (DHEF) by Crawford and Serhal (2020) defines the digital determinants of health as

> individuals' access to digital resources, use of these resources for health seeking, digital health literacy, beliefs about the potential help or harm of digital health care, values and cultural preferences regarding the use of digital resources, and integration of digital resources into community and health infrastructure.

Another proposed framework for advancing Digital Health equity, proposed by Richardson et al. (2022), is structured across multiple domains, including biological factors, behavioural determinants, the physical and built environment, the sociocultural environment, and the healthcare system. These domains align with the socioecological model, emphasising a multilevel approach to understanding health disparities. Social Determinants of Health (SDH) are predominantly represented in the domains of the physical/built environment, the sociocultural environment, and the healthcare system, reflecting their significant influence on health outcomes. This framework adapts the National Institute on Aging (NIA) disparities model by incorporating the healthcare system as a distinct domain, acknowledging its critical role in health disparities. This adaptation, known as the National Institute on Minority Health and Health Disparities (NIMHD) Research Framework, underscores the interconnectedness of various determinants and the importance of addressing systemic factors to achieve health equity in Digital Health initiatives (Table 6.1).

Digital Health: Navigating Challenges and Advancing Equity

Digital Health offers considerable potential to reduce disparities in healthcare access and delivery; however, several long-standing challenges must first be addressed to fully realise its benefits. Although there is a global increase in smartphone coverage and use, not everyone has access, particularly people living in rural areas, where poor internet connectivity and unreliable access to electricity impede the adoption of DHTs. Additionally, cost poses a substantial obstacle, as the high expense of devices and services disproportionately

TABLE 6.1 Framework for Digital Health Equity from the Lenses of the Domains and Levels of Influence. Adopted from the National Institute on Minority Health and Health Disparities Research Framework Expanded for Digital Health Equity

Domain/Level of Influence	Individual	Interpersonal	Community	Societal
Biological	Biological vulnerability and mechanisms	Caregiver–child interaction, family microbiome	Community illness exposure, herd immunity	Sanitation, immunisation, pathogen exposure
Behavioural	Health behaviours, coping strategies	Family, school, work functioning	Community functioning, community resources	Policies and laws
Physical/Built Environment	Personal environment	Household, school, work environment	Community environment, community resources	Societal structure
Digital Environment	Digital literacy, digital self-efficacy, technology access, attitudes towards use	Implicit tech bias, interdependence (e.g., shared devices), patient-tech-clinician relationship	Community infrastructure, healthcare infrastructure, community tech norms, community partners	Tech policy, data standards, design standards, social norms and ideologies, algorithmic bias
Sociocultural Environment	Sociodemographics, limited English proficiency, cultural identity, response to discrimination	Social networks, family/peer norms, interpersonal discrimination	Community norms, local structural discrimination	Social norms, societal structural discrimination
Healthcare System	Insurance coverage, health literacy, treatment preferences	Patient-clinician relationship, medical decision-making	Availability of services	Quality of care, healthcare policies

affects low-income populations. The issue of Digital Health literacy further complicates the situation, with many individuals lacking the necessary skills to navigate and utilise Digital Health tools effectively. Moreover, concerns regarding data privacy and the equitable safeguarding of patient information must be prioritised to foster trust and inclusivity in Digital Health initiatives.

To advance Digital Health equity, several opportunities can be pursued. These include expanding public-private partnerships to enhance infrastructure development and improving the affordability of Digital Health solutions. Culturally appropriate interventions, developed through meaningful co-creation with end users, can ensure that Digital Health tools not only are accessible and relevant to diverse populations but also leverage user-centred design approaches, which is explored in detail in Chapter 7. Finally, the implementation of policies mandating equity-driven standards for Digital Health technologies is crucial in establishing a framework for fairness and inclusivity in their development and deployment.

DIGITAL LITERACY AS A DETERMINANT OF HEALTH

As the role of DHTs becomes increasingly significant in healthcare, individuals must have sufficient and adequate digital skills. *Digital literacy* is a term that refers to these digital skills and is the collective ability to find and apply digital information and consciously make use of technology (López et al., 2023).

This need for specific skills to navigate healthcare systems and manage health through digital resources has given rise to the concept of "Digital Health literacy". Several definitions of Digital Health literacy have been proposed, starting with Norman and Skinner's conceptualisation of eHealth literacy as "the ability to seek, find, understand, and appraise health information from electronic sources and apply the knowledge gained to addressing or solving a health problem". More recently, this initial concept has been expanded and broadly defined as "the capacity to translate health knowledge acquired from digital environments" (Ban et al., 2024). Not all individuals have the same level of Digital Health literacy, which is influenced by sociodemographic, economic, and cultural factors (Estrela et al., 2023).

Digital Health literacy has been recognised as a key social determinant of health—in parallel to socioeconomic status, income, education, age, gender, ethnicity, and race (López et al., 2023)—and it plays a critical role in enabling equitable access to Digital Health services. On the one hand, digital innovations have the potential to improve not only self-care and home-based care but also health outcomes. On the other hand, as health systems become increasingly reliant on DHTs, disparities between those with adequate digital skills and those without tend to increase. Individuals who cannot access Digital Health tools, who do not know how to use such tools, or who do not recognise their importance are less likely to use and benefit from Digital Health innovations. Moreover, low digital literacy can exacerbate existing barriers and vulnerabilities since it substantially interacts with other social determinants of health. Through this intersectionality of disadvantages, underserved populations who already experience inequality in healthcare (e.g., rural populations, older individuals, minorities, and persons with disabilities) are at a greater risk of experiencing low Digital Health literacy and being further digitally excluded.

The recognition of digital literacy as a social determinant of health and its fundamental role in promoting health equity has led to the development of different interventions that aim to improve Digital Health literacy and empower individuals to make informed health decisions. Educational and training initiatives are the most often reported initiatives to address poor Digital Health literacy. Examples of such initiatives include massive open online courses, university training in Digital Health through tutoring, and online video-based portal training (López et al., 2023). In the US, an on-line video-based training program was developed to explain how to use the on-line patient portal MYSFHEALTH. The training program was tested in two clinics of the San Francisco Health Network among vulnerable patients with more than one chronic disease, a low socioeconomic status, and limited health literacy. The training program increased Digital Health literacy over time and moderately increased portal use in the follow-up months. The participants self-reported improvement in their portal skills and more confidence using the patient portal (Lyles, et al., 2018).

It is vital to raise awareness of the importance of Digital Health literacy for better health outcomes and to recognise digital literacy as a contemporary determinant of health. The quest for more inclusive DHTs to address the digital divide depends on improving access to Digital Health information and tools for people with low digital literacy, which should be a social and public health priority.

THE DIGITAL DIVIDE

The digital divide refers to the gap between those who have access to information and communication technologies (ICTs) and those who do not. Several key factors contribute to this divide, including socioeconomic factors such as affordability of devices and internet connectivity, geographic limitations particularly in rural and remote areas, and a lack of digital literacy skills.

The digital divide aggravates existing health disparities by limiting access to essential DHTs. These disparities are particularly pronounced among marginalised populations including low-income countries, women, the elderly, migrants, refugees, and rural populations. For instance, a 2023 Global System for Mobile Communications Association (GSMA) report highlights that although smartphone ownership among women in low- and middle-income countries (LMICs) has increased, a significant proportion still lacks access. Another report by the International Telecommunication Union (ITU) indicates that rural populations in LMICs often have lower rates of internet access than urban areas. Lower levels of education and exposure to technology in rural communities can further hinder the adoption of Digital Health tools.

"Digital redlining", a modern-day echo of historical redlining practices, worsens the digital divide by systematically denying certain communities access to essential digital infrastructure and services. This discriminatory practice often targets marginalised communities based on socioeconomic status, race, and ethnicity. When communities are redlined, they are deprived of high-speed internet access, affordable data plans, and reliable digital devices. This lack of connectivity has far-reaching consequences for health equity. Individuals in these communities may struggle to access critical health information, schedule appointments, or participate in telehealth consultations. They may also be unable to download health apps or access online health portals, limiting their ability to manage chronic conditions and make informed health decisions.

Geographic accessibility is also a major obstacle, with rural areas often lacking the necessary infrastructure investment due to low population density, challenging terrain, and high deployment costs. Broadband plans can be prohibitively expensive for low-income households, limiting access for a substantial portion of the population. Additionally, digital literacy skills are often lacking, which hinders the effective use of the internet and DHTs even when they are available. According to the ITU, 94% of the world's unconnected population resides in LMICs (Delaporte et al, 2022). The GSMA reports that adults in rural areas of LMICs are 33% less likely to use mobile internet than their urban counterparts.

Device access remains a significant barrier to DHTs, particularly in LMICs. The affordability of devices such as smartphones, tablets, and computers can be prohibitive for many people. This significantly limits access to essential health information, telemedicine consultations, and other Digital Health tools. These disparities highlight the urgent need to address these challenges and bridge the digital divide in LMICs.

Mitigating the Digital Divide

To bridge the digital divide and improve health equity, a multifaceted approach is essential. Expanding broadband access to underserved areas, particularly rural and low-income communities, is crucial. Investing in infrastructure and implementing affordable internet plans can ensure equitable access to

Digital Health services. Additionally, providing affordable devices and digital literacy training can empower individuals to navigate the digital world effectively. Furthermore, developing culturally and linguistically appropriate Digital Health tools can help overcome language barriers and improve health outcomes for diverse populations. Mobile health solutions, such as telemedicine and health apps, can reach underserved communities, especially those in remote areas. Policy interventions, including subsidies for internet access and digital literacy programs, can further support digital equity and reduce health disparities.

CASE STUDY   BACKGROUND HEALTHEMOVE

Displaced individuals, including refugees and undocumented migrants, often face exclusion from national healthcare programs. They typically receive limited, fragmented emergency care due to political and logistical challenges. Their mobility further disrupts continuity of care, especially because of the lack of access to previous medical records, leading to delays in treatment and suboptimal healthcare, which exacerbate health disparities.

An opportunity for change lies in the increasing adoption of smartphones among refugees and migrants. Smartphone adoption gives this group the opportunity to benefit significantly from Digital Health interventions.

In this case, we turn to the experience of the Netherlands where there has been considerable investment and lawmaking to provide an electronic personal health record to every citizen, but only a very limited group of citizens is using it. However, people on the move such as refugees and undocumented migrants might find it very beneficial to develop and use their own electronic personal health record.

Developing and Implementing the Pilot Initiative "HealthEmove"

HealthEmove is an electronic personal health record (EPHR) for mobile populations. It uses the software from Patients Know Best (PKB), one of the largest EPHR providers in the world. As the CEO of PKB is a descendant of refugees himself and has a rare disease that he frequently had to explain to new healthcare providers, the company supports HealthEmove to develop and implement an EPHR for people on the move.

Central to the philosophy of HealthEmove is the principle of individual autonomy and individual empowerment in healthcare. For displaced populations, fragmented and inaccessible medical histories often create critical gaps in care. By placing control of medical records directly in the hands of individuals, HealthEmove enables them to

- Enhance Autonomy: Maintain and manage their health records independently;
- Improve Continuity of Care: Share medical histories with new healthcare providers, reducing duplicative diagnostics and improving treatment outcomes; and
- Foster Trust in Care: Encourage individuals to actively participate in their healthcare decisions.

HealthEmove is a web-based health record in 22 languages and provides a secure Digital Health platform, in line with the General Data Protection Regulation (GDPR), tailored to the needs of "people on the move". It bridges the gap in healthcare continuity by providing individuals with ownership and control of their medical data. HealthEmove is developed and implemented through a co-creative process with affected communities. Users can securely store and share a range of health data, including diagnoses, medications, uploaded PDFs, and images, in a "safe digital vault". Both individuals and healthcare providers can contribute to the record, with transparency regarding who entered specific data. No user can alter entries made by others. Individuals are encouraged and educated to add any available medical information and continually update their health records.

Lessons Learned

The pilot initiative in 2024 among 170 users in Amsterdam highlights both successes and challenges. Participants were overall very positive about the concept of getting access to—and ownership of—their own medical information. In addition to medical documents that were added by UDM themselves, other documents such as social data were stored in the tool. With the support of community leaders, participants often trusted the security of the tool.

Digital exclusivity remained a concern, particularly for elderly individuals and those without smartphones or email addresses or with limited digital skills. To address this, HealthEmove implemented in-person workshops, so-called walk-in days, and tailored support that even includes in some situations setting up a new email account.

In general, one of the main dilemmas is striking the right balance between privacy and data security. The current platform requires two-factor authentication (2FA) using a Google Authenticator application, in line with Dutch regulations. However, downloading and installing this application was often considered a key challenge. Some participants wondered if the tool can be developed to run like Facebook: opening an app that immediately shows the medical history and removing the 2FA. This shows that not all individuals are aware of the importance of secure data protection.

Scaling HealthEmove

HealthEmove exemplifies how tailored Digital Health solutions can bridge the divide for vulnerable groups, improving both health outcomes and system efficiency. The initiative plans to expand across Europe, aiming to create a unified Digital Health platform accessible to all individuals, regardless of their migratory status or origin. By leveraging partnerships with organisations such as Patients Know Best and local healthcare networks, HealthEmove envisions a future where no one is excluded from quality healthcare due to frequent mobility.

ALGORITHMIC BIAS IN DIGITAL HEALTH

The increasing integration of artificial intelligence (AI) and machine learning (ML) in Digital Health systems has the potential to revolutionise Primary Care. However, as these technologies become more pervasive, concerns about algorithmic bias and its implications for health equity grow. Algorithmic bias occurs when AI or ML systems produce results that are systematically prejudiced because of flawed data sets, model design, or implementation contexts.

Key Implications of Algorithmic Bias

Algorithmic bias can significantly exacerbate health inequities (Table 6.2). An obvious example of algorithmic bias occurred in a health risk prediction tool used in the US healthcare system by insurers. Researchers found that the algorithm disproportionately prioritised white patients over black patients for high-risk care management programs (Obermeyer, 2019). The bias stemmed from the algorithm's reliance on healthcare spending as a proxy for health needs, overlooking systemic disparities in healthcare access and utilisation among black patients.

AI-driven diagnostic tools rely on training data that may not represent diverse populations. Inequitable diagnostic performance can exacerbate existing health disparities, particularly for underrepresented populations. Skin lesion detection algorithms trained predominantly on lighter skin tones may underperform on darker skin tones, leading to missed or delayed diagnoses of melanoma (Chen RJ, 2023). Cardiovascular risk assessment tools have been

TABLE 6.2 Major Patterns of Algorithmic Bias in Health

Pattern of Bias	Description
Data Set Bias	AI systems trained on incomplete or non-representative data sets may generate outputs that favour certain populations while marginalising others.
Model Bias	Bias introduced through model design, where the assumptions that underpin the algorithms fail to account for the diversity of user populations.
Deployment Bias	This refers to the systematic disparity that arises when Digital Health interventions, such as eHealth technologies or AI-driven tools, are deployed in ways that disproportionately benefit certain groups over others.

Source: Author, 2024.

found to overestimate or underestimate risk in racial and ethnic minorities due to underrepresentation in the data sets used for training (Wong ND, 2022).

Predictive analytics in eHealth, such as risk stratification for chronic diseases, often use socioeconomic and historical health data. These data sets can reflect systemic inequities, such as disparities in access to healthcare or historical discrimination. Predictive models may inadvertently penalise individuals from low-income or marginalised communities by assigning them lower priority for interventions.

Additionally, personalised medicine aims to tailor treatments to individual genetic, environmental, and lifestyle factors. However, most genomic data used in AI-driven research come from individuals of European descent, which limits the applicability of these models to other populations. This also limits the potential of personalised medicine to achieve its promise of inclusivity and effectiveness. Pharmacogenomic algorithms may not accurately predict drug efficacy or safety in patients from underrepresented genetic backgrounds.

Addressing Algorithmic Bias in eHealth

To mitigate algorithmic bias in eHealth, AI models must be trained on diverse data sets that accurately represent global populations, including variations in gender, age, ethnicity, and socioeconomic backgrounds. Regular audits of these data sets are essential to identify and correct biases at the source. Integrating fairness metrics into model development will help evaluate performance across different demographic groups and ensure that algorithms provide equitable outcomes for all users. Additionally, making AI models interpretable enhances accountability and trust, allowing stakeholders to understand how decisions are made. Collaboration with community groups and healthcare providers is vital to ensure that algorithms are tailored to meet the specific needs of local populations. Finally, implementing mechanisms to monitor algorithmic performance and address unintended consequences post-deployment is crucial to monitor inequities and mitigate them during deployment.

FUTURE DIRECTIONS IN POLICY AND REGULATION FOR DIGITAL HEALTH EQUITY

The future of Digital Health equity in Primary Care is intrinsically linked to innovative policies and regulatory frameworks that address systemic inequities and the digital divide. Legislative measures like the 21st Century Cures Act (2016) have demonstrated the importance of creating and enabling an environment for Digital Health by mandating interoperability, empowering patients with access to their health data, and fostering innovation through supportive funding and research policies. These changes help break down silos in healthcare data and enable seamless sharing across providers and technologies, which is vital for delivering equitable, patient-centred care (DeSalvo et al., 2021).

Addressing the digital divide is essential for reducing disparities in access to Digital Health services. Geographic disparities, such as the lack of broadband infrastructure in rural areas, and economic barriers, including the affordability of devices and internet plans, remain significant hurdles. Policies that expand broadband access, provide subsidies for devices, and ensure telehealth reimbursement equity can help bridge this gap. For instance, federal initiatives such as the Federal Communications Commission's Rural Digital Opportunity Fund in the US and individual state-level programs aimed at subsidising broadband access demonstrate the potential of targeted investments to transform connectivity in underserved regions (Park et al., 2021).

Inclusive design in Digital Health technologies is another critical policy direction. Regulatory frameworks must enforce diversity in clinical trials to ensure Digital Health tools that are co-developed, tested and validated at all stages across varied populations. Accessibility standards, such as compliance with the Americans with Disabilities Act (ADA) in Digital Health platforms, and the incorporation of culturally sensitive and linguistically appropriate tools are equally important. These measures ensure that Digital Health innovations cater to diverse populations, including those often left behind by technological advancements, such as older adults, non-English speakers, and people with disabilities (Hoffman & Podgurski, 2021).

Data privacy and algorithmic equity are also pivotal concerns in the Digital Health landscape. Policies that strengthen privacy laws, such as the General

Data Protection Regulation (GDPR) in Europe, can serve as models to protect sensitive health data. Transparency in algorithm development and ongoing evaluation of their performance across diverse populations are key regulatory priorities (Hernandez-Boussard et al., 2020).

Global perspectives offer valuable insights. For example, India's Ayushman Bharat Digital Mission integrates Digital Health tools into its universal healthcare system, leveraging mobile health technologies to reach underserved populations. Similarly, the European Union's Digital Health Strategy stresses the importance of interoperability and data security within its multi-country framework and provides a roadmap for balancing innovation with equity and trust (European Commission, 2022).

Finally, fostering public-private partnerships can play a transformative role in accelerating the adoption of equitable Digital Health solutions. Incentives for private companies to invest in underserved areas or co-develop culturally tailored tools with public health systems can drive sustainable progress. Through these collaborative efforts, stakeholders can address gaps in funding, technology, and access to create a truly inclusive Digital Health ecosystem.

KEY MESSAGES

- Inequities in Digital Health access worsen existing health disparities among marginalised populations, necessitating inclusive solutions.
- The digital divide refers to the gap between those who have access to information and communication technologies and those who do not have access. The key factors that contribute to this divide include the affordability of devices, access to internet connectivity, geographic limitations, particularly in rural and remote areas, and a lack of digital literacy skills.
- Digital literacy is now a recognised social determinant of health. Enhancing digital skills is vital for bridging the digital divide and addressing pre-existing, current, and future health inequities.
- The co-creation of inclusive Digital Health initiatives specifically aimed at marginalised populations, such as mobile populations, can reduce health disparities and minimise the digital divide.
- Inclusive data training and transparency in AI systems are essential to avoid exacerbating health disparities. Expanding public-private partnerships and fostering culturally and linguistically appropriate interventions are pivotal.

NOTE: ChatGPT was used for idea generation and language improvement.

REFERENCES

1. World Health Organization. *Global strategy on digital health 2020–2025.* Geneva: World Health Organization; 2021. Licence: CC BY-NC-SA 3.0 IGO.

2. Crawford A, Serhal E. Digital health equity and COVID-19: the innovation curve cannot reinforce the social gradient of health. *J Med Internet Res.* 2020 Jun 2;22(6):e19361. https://doi.org/10.2196/19361. PMID: 32452816; PMCID: PMC7268667.

3. Kaihlanen AM, Virtanen L, Buchert U, et al. Towards digital health equity: a qualitative study of the challenges experienced by vulnerable groups in using digital health services in the COVID-19 era. *BMC Health Serv Res.* 2022;22:188. https://doi.org/10.1186/s12913-022-07584-4.

4. Richardson S, Lawrence K, Schoenthaler AM, et al. A framework for digital health equity. *NPJ Digit Med.* 2022;5:119. https://doi.org/10.1038/s41746-022-00663-0.

5. Groom LL, Schoenthaler AM, Mann DM, et al. Construction of the digital health equity-focused implementation research conceptual model—bridging the divide between equity-focused digital health and implementation research. *PLoS Digit Health.* 2024;3(5):e0000509. https://doi.org/10.1371/journal.pdig.

6. Ban S, Kim Y, Seomun G. Digital health literacy: a concept analysis. *Digit Health.* 2024 Oct 7. https://doi.org/10.1177/20552076241287894. PMID: 39381807; PMCID: PMC11459536.

7. Estrela M, Semedo G, Roque F, et al. Sociodemographic determinants of digital health literacy: a systematic review and meta-analysis. *Int J Med Inform.* 2023 Sep;177:105124. https://doi.org/10.1016/j.ijmedinf.2023.105124. Epub 2023 Jun 10. PMID: 37329766.

8. Lyles CR, Tieu L, Sarkar U, et al. A randomized trial to train vulnerable primary care patients to use a patient portal. *J Am Board Fam Med.* 2019 Mar–Apr;32(2):248–58. https://doi.org/10.3122/jabfm.2019.02.180263. PMID: 30850461; PMCID: PMC6647853.

9. Arias López MDP, Ong BA, Borrat Frigola X, et al. Digital literacy as a new determinant of health: a scoping review. *PLoS Digit Health.* 2023 Oct 12;2(10):e0000279. https://doi.org/10.1371/journal.pdig.0000279. PMID: 37824584; PMCID: PMC10569540.

10. Chen RJ, Wang JJ, Williamson DFK, et al. Algorithmic fairness in artificial intelligence for medicine and healthcare. *Nat Biomed Eng.* 2023 Jun;7(6):719–42. https://doi.org/10.1038/s41551-023-01056-8. Epub 2023 Jun 28. PMID: 37380750; PMCID: PMC10632090.

11. Obermeyer Z, Powers B, Vogeli C, et al. Dissecting racial bias in an algorithm used to manage the health of populations. *Science.* 2019 Oct 25;366(6464):447–53. https://doi.org/10.1126/science.aax2342. PMID: 31649194.

12. Wong ND, Budoff MJ, Ferdinand K, et al. Atherosclerotic cardiovascular disease risk assessment: an American society for preventive cardiology clinical practice statement. *Am J Prev Cardiol.* 2022 Mar 15;10:100335. https://doi.org/10.1016/j.ajpc.2022.100335. PMID: 35342890; PMCID: PMC8943256.

CHAPTER 7

User-Centred Design and User Experiences with Digital Health

Geva Greenfield, Ana Rita Luz,
Boon How Chew, Kam Cheong Wong,
and Cristina Jácome

USER EXPERIENCE (UX) IN DIGITAL PRIMARY CARE

Understanding User Experience (UX) in the Context of Healthcare Settings

Primary Care is the first point of care in most countries and the main route of interaction with the healthcare systems for most patients. Hence, a satisfying patient experience and a positive healthcare professional (HCP) experience are crucial for improved health outcomes, satisfaction, and efficient use of resources. The UX paradigm, which prioritises the central role of users in system interactions and processes, aligns closely with contemporary healthcare approaches such as person-centred care, integrated care, care co-designed with patients, and patient empowerment.

To understand what UX in Digital Health means, we first need to understand the specific context of receiving and providing healthcare—i.e., the needs and preferences of those seeking care and of those providing care. In healthcare settings, UX is not purely about convenience or efficiency but also about people's own health and safety. In its essence, measurement of UX in Primary Care digital tools is no different than UX measurement in other industries. Similar tools and techniques such as the analysis of usage data, observations, emotion assessments, focus groups, affinity diagrams, storyboarding, and card sorting can be applied (Still et al., 2017). There is also a notion that the existing terminology (e.g., user experience, usability, and participatory design) is not adequate to apply 'as is' for UX and usability work in healthcare contexts and needs to be adapted accordingly (Melonçon, 2017).

Challenges in Achieving an Optimal User Experience

Many healthcare systems, traditionally built alongside the biomedical model, still prioritise achieving health outcomes in a timely manner over patient experience. Tax-funded public healthcare systems and privately funded, insurance-based healthcare systems often focus on meeting patient demand in a timely and cost-effective manner. Developing a good user experience (UX) is often perceived as 'nice to have' but not a top priority. In recent decades, there has been a shift toward prioritising patient experience; however, this mindset change will take time to be fully embraced and embedded into healthcare services.

The fragmented and complex nature of healthcare systems, Primary Care, secondary care, tertiary care, social care, and mental health—all operating in different organisational cultures that implement different processes and use different information technology systems—is a massive challenge for designers. Strict compliance regulations require protection of the sensitive nature of health data and introduce an additional challenge to optimised UX. Other common challenges involve engaging users in healthcare design and catering to the conflicting needs of diverse user groups, particularly the elderly and those with low digital literacy, using the same product or platform.

Adopting Digital Health technology across different Primary Care sites and institutions can face several barriers that hinder optimal experience. These challenges span psychological, technical, and operational aspects and often require tailored solutions to ensure an effective integration (Kim, 2024). One major challenge is that primary HCPs may find it hard to see how the new technology fits into their care models. Additionally, digital tools designed for specific institutions often do not adapt well to different Primary Care settings. Technical challenges often come from differences in digital systems between institutions. Many Primary Care facilities lack the resources needed to set up and maintain Digital Health tools, so technologies that are easy to use and require minimal support are more appealing. A lack of standardisation across healthcare settings can also have negative impacts on UX; design systems that are interoperable allow a smoother transition across different digital platforms and can improve UX.

Introducing Digital Health tools can also cause worries about disrupting current workflows, especially if they add extra administrative tasks. To avoid this, tools should combine clinical and administrative functions on one platform, cutting down the need for extra systems and improving efficiency.

Complicated setups and long onboarding times can slow implementation and discourage use. A 'ready-to-use' approach with minimal setup can make adoption quicker and transitions smoother for healthcare teams.

Digital literacy and trust issues can also be a challenge for optimal UX. As Fitzpatrick (2023) emphasises, information must be presented in a clear and actionable manner and consider the varying literacy levels across different populations. Digital Health literacy plays a critical role that empowers patients to effectively engage with technology and leverage digital tools to manage their health. Patients are no longer passive recipients of care; instead, they are active partners in their health journey. This collaborative relationship ensures that care is both personalised and effective. Transparency and ethical implementation remain central to building trust in Digital Health tools for both patients and HCPs.

USER-CENTRED DESIGN (UCD) IN DIGITAL PRIMARY CARE
Definitions and Principles of User-Centred Design (UCD)

As the name suggests, UCD prioritises the user rather than the technology or product itself. It involves designing solutions that are tailored to users' needs, goals, and preferences, ensuring a more intuitive and effective experience. Conceptually, UCD interacts with other related concepts, such as user experience, usability, and human-computer interaction. UCD encompasses a set of design principles, including proximity, visibility, visual feedback, visual prominence, hierarchy, and mental models and metaphors. UCD emphasises early, frequent, and iterative user engagement throughout the design process. It ensures alignment with real-world usage contexts, prioritises simplicity, empowers users with greater control, considers emotional design factors, and incorporates continuous iterative testing for improvement (Still and Crane, 2017). However, UCD is more than a set of practical design principles; it is an approach that prioritises the user's goals, needs, preferences, and capacities.

Designing effective Digital Health tools requires a user-centred approach to confirm that they are practical, trustworthy, and suitable for healthcare settings (European Commission, 2019). This involves key steps, from design to deployment and ongoing evaluation, and creating tools that meet the needs of patients, providers, and stakeholders. Each step includes best practices for user engagement, ethics, regulations, and system integration that ensure that the tools meet technical standards while improving care delivery, safety, and access (STANDING Together, 2023; European Commission, 2019; Fehr, 2024).

One important step is defining the tool's purpose, target users, and expected outcomes while ensuring that ethical considerations, bias mitigation, and privacy safeguards are in place (Kwong, 2023; STANDING Together, 2023). Early stakeholder engagement through interviews, surveys, and observational studies is critical to gather insights and to confirm that the tool meets diverse needs, accounting for geographical, linguistic, and digital skill variations. Creating user personas helps to represent different segments of the target audience, guiding the subsequent design phases. Furthermore, a thorough review of policies ensures compliance with guidelines related to autonomy, privacy, transparency, and environmental impacts.

Once user insights are gathered, the next steps generally include ideation and concept development, where potential solutions are brainstormed and prioritised based on user needs. Prototyping comes next, which involves the creation of low-fidelity sketches and high-fidelity interactive models to visualise the solution. When the digital tool includes an AI component, high data quality and model integrity are equally essential during the development phase (STANDING Together, 2023). This begins with data collection and preparation and involves cleaning and preprocessing to address missing values, outliers, and inconsistencies (Kwong, 2023). Subsequently, exploratory data analysis helps to assess data characteristics and quality (Collins, 2024). To confirm the tool's relevance, model selection and feature engineering must suit the Digital Health tool, balancing performance, interpretability, and scalability. Moreover, training and testing the model on separate datasets are essential to ensure accuracy, generalisability, and reliability under diverse conditions (Collins, 2024; Kwong, 2023).

Once a prototype is ready, it is essential to conduct usability testing sessions with real users to gather feedback. This process should be iterative, involving repeated testing and refinement until the design aligns with user expectations. Successful deployment builds on the aforementioned foundations and emphasises smooth integration and thorough user training. Digital tools must align with existing clinical workflows and patient care pathways to minimise disruptions. Comprehensive training for clinical staff, administrators, and patients fosters trust and ensures effective use by clearly explaining the tool's purpose, functions, and limitations.

Finally, the post-deployment phase requires a focus on continuous improvement and accountability. Regular reviews of the digital tool's performance are necessary to measure its impact on health outcomes, service quality, and patient satisfaction while identifying opportunities for refinement (European Commission, 2019; Fehr, 2024). Safety monitoring and clear error-reporting protocols are vital to address risks and maintain user trust. Sustainability and usability evaluations, including ecosystem assessments and cost analyses, ensure that the tool remains practical and adaptable over time (Kwong, 2023). Governance policies must further confirm responsible use, risk management, and the availability of rollback options if needed. Continuous stakeholder engagement ensures that the tool evolves with user feedback, fostering trust and shared accountability throughout its lifecycle.

User-Centred Design Cases in Primary Care

Three examples were selected to showcase the iterative UCD process in the development of Digital Health tools.

Tierney et al. (2023) focused on design iterations to refine a software application, aiming to improve diet discussions between clinicians and patients in Primary Care. Through three iterations of design and review, there was substantial evolution of the program's content, format, and flow of information, which involved 'tuning' the information according to clinicians and patient perceptions for optimal dietary goal setting. Korpershoek et al. (2020) described the UCD process for an mHealth intervention aimed at enhancing the self-management of chronic obstructive pulmonary disease (COPD) that comprised four phases: (1) background analysis and design conceptualisation, (2) alpha usability testing, (3) iterative software development, and (4) field usability testing. By following a UCD process and involving extensive stakeholder engagement, an mHealth intervention was developed that met the needs and preferences of patients with COPD, is likely to be used by these patients, and has a high potential to be effective in reducing the exacerbation impact. Finally, Kirkwood et al. (2024) utilised ethnographic observations and semi-structured interviews to design an mHealth tool for gestational diabetes, integrating a clinical dashboard with a patient-facing app, which received positive feedback from users for effectively meeting their needs (Kirkwood et al., 2024). Together, these examples illustrate the application of UCD methodologies in creating tailored Digital Health solutions that address the specific needs of patients and healthcare professionals (HCPs).

IMPACT OF DIGITAL HEALTH ON PATIENT-CENTREDNESS

Patient-centred care is the cornerstone of a sustained patient-HCP relationship and ensures that an individual's specific health needs and desired outcomes guide all healthcare decisions and quality measures. Through this holistic perspective, primary healthcare providers need to build trust and understanding, cultivate sustained relationships that honor patient autonomy and promote meaningful collaboration, and pave the way for more personalised care.

As healthcare evolves, Digital Health technologies have been playing a fundamental role in transforming patient-centred care, making it more personalised, accessible, and effective. Digital Health technologies enhance access to care, offer personalised health insights, and improve communication between patients and providers. For instance, patient portals linked to electronic health records can offer individuals access to their medical history, test results, and care plans, ensuring continuity of care. Telehealth platforms may allow patients to consult with HCPs from the comfort of their homes, which overcomes barriers such as distance and mobility issues. Mobile applications and online scheduling systems make healthcare more convenient, enabling patients to connect with HCPs on their own terms. Wearables, health trackers, and patient portals empower individuals to monitor their health in real time, which offers valuable insights into their conditions and encourages proactive management (Leonardsen, 2023). These technologies also enable better clinical decision-making by providing HCPs with real-time patient data, supporting timely interventions and collaboration across disciplines (Fitzpatrick, 2023).

Therefore, incorporating patient perspectives is essential when evaluating the effectiveness and usability of Digital Health solutions (Bronneke, 2023). To measure patient-centred outcomes and the device's usability, the evaluation methods should be personalised for users. One example is the use of visualisation tools to assess patients' asthma symptoms using a visual analogue scale and daily electronic asthma scores, which have been reported to optimise treatment and improve symptoms and quality of life (Sousa-Pinto, 2023). The technology acceptance model (TAM) has been developed and applied to evaluate users' perceptions of usefulness and ease of use, which predict their adoption of technology. However, the TAM does not evaluate the technology or device's time efficiency. In contrast, the International Organization of Standardization (ISO) includes time efficiency, device reliability, and user satisfaction in usability evaluations. Both the TAM and ISO guidelines can be used to evaluate Digital Health initiatives. To streamline the evaluation, patient experience, time efficiency and device reliability approaches can be incorporated into the TAM (Wong, 2024). A patient-centredness evaluation can be further explored in qualitative interviews. The patient's context and agency (i.e., ability and willingness to use Digital Health innovations) must be included in the evaluation. The critical realism approach (i.e., what works for whom in what circumstances and how to enable patients to adopt the innovation) allows for an in-depth assessment. Mixed-methods analysis (e.g., integrating qualitative evaluation with quantitative assessments) provides additional nuance to evaluations, generating insights on the underlying mechanisms of the effective use of Digital Health, its enablers, and its barriers through a patient-centred lens (Wong, 2024).

KEY MESSAGES

- By prioritising the needs and experiences of both patients and HCPs, we can create tools that effectively enhance patient-centred care and improve user experience (UX).
- The implementation of Digital Health technologies presents significant challenges to user experience that originate from

suboptimal digital literacy, varying healthcare infrastructures, and concerns about workload and trust.
- User-centred design (UCD) is an iterative approach that encompasses user research, prototyping, and ongoing evaluation to ensure that solutions seamlessly integrate into existing workflows and that diverse user needs are addressed.

NOTE: GPT-4o was used for paragraphs and ideas synthesis, readability and language improvement.

REFERENCES

Brönneke JB, Herr A, Reif S, et al. Dynamic HTA for digital health solutions: opportunities and challenges for patient-centered evaluation. *Int J Technol Assess Health Care.* 2023;39(1):e72. https://doi.org/10.1017/S0266462323002726.

Collins GS, Moons KGM, Dhiman P, et al. TRIPOD+AI statement: updated guidance for reporting clinical prediction models that use regression or machine learning methods. *BMJ.* 2024;e078378. Cited 2024 May 2. Available from: https://www.bmj.com/lookup/doi/10.1136/bmj-2023-078378.

Fehr J, Citro B, Malpani R, Lippert C, et al. A trustworthy AI reality-check: the lack of transparency of artificial intelligence products in healthcare. *Front Digit Health.* 2024;6:1267290. Cited 2024 Mar 20. Available from: https://www.frontiersin.org/articles/10.3389/fdgth.2024.1267290/full.

Fitzpatrick PJ. Improving health literacy using the power of digital communications to achieve better health outcomes for patients and practitioners. *Front Digit Health.* 2023 Nov 17;5:1264780. https://doi.org/10.3389/fdgth.2023.1264780. PMID: 38046643; PMCID: PMC10693297.

Kim GYK, Rostosky R, Bishop FK, et al. The adaptation of a single institution diabetes care platform into a nationally available turnkey solution. *NPJ Digit Med.* 2024;7:311. https://doi.org/10.1038/s41746-024-01319-x.

Kirkwood JR, Dickson J, Stevens M, et al. The user-centered design of a clinical dashboard and patient-facing app for gestational diabetes. *J Diabetes Sci Technol.* 2024 Nov 29. https://doi.org/10.1177/19322968241301792.

Korpershoek YJG, Hermsen S, Schoonhoven L, et al. User-centered design of a mobile health intervention to enhance exacerbation-related self-management in patients with chronic obstructive pulmonary disease (Copilot): mixed methods study. *J Med Internet Res.* 2020 Jun 15;22(6):e15449. https://doi.org/10.2196/15449.

Kwong JCC, Khondker A, Lajkosz K, et al. APPRAISE-AI tool for quantitative evaluation of AI studies for clinical decision support. *JAMA Netw Open.* 2023;6(9):e2335377. Cited 2024 Mar 20. Available from: https://jamanetwork.com/journals/jamanetworkopen/fullarticle/2809841.

Leonardsen AL, Bååth C, Helgesen AK, et al. Person-centeredness in digital primary healthcare services: a scoping review. *Healthcare (Basel).* 2023 May 1;11(9):1296. https://doi.org/10.3390/healthcare11091296. PMID: 37174838; PMCID: PMC10178010.

Sousa-Pinto B, Jácome C, Pereira AM, et al. Development and validation of an electronic daily control score for asthma (e-DASTHMA): a real-world direct patient data study. *Lancet Digit Health.* 2023 Apr 1;5(4):e227–38. Epub 2023 Mar 3. https://doi.org/10.1016/S2589-7500(23)00020-1.

The STANDING Together Collaboration. Recommendations for diversity, inclusivity, and generalisability in artificial intelligence health technologies and health datasets. 2023. Available from: https://zenodo.org/doi/10.5281/zenodo.10048356.

Tierney WM, Henning JM, Altillo BS, et al. User-centered design of a clinical tool for shared decision-making about diet in primary care. *J Gen Intern Med.* 2023 Feb;38(3):715–26.

Wong KC. *Atrial fibrillation screening in the community: an integrated continual care approach.* PhD dissertation, University of Sydney; 2024. Available from: https://ses.library.usyd.edu.au/handle/2123/33258.

CHAPTER 8

Implementing Digital Health Solutions in Primary Care

Geronimo Jimenez, Marise Kasteleyn,
Niels Chavannes, Raluca Zoiţanu,
and Ahmed Alboksmaty

INTEGRATING DIGITAL HEALTH INTO PRIMARY CARE

Digital Health offers an exciting, game-changing path forward, empowering Primary Care to rise above contemporary challenges and redefine its role as a cornerstone of health and well-being.[1] However, Digital Health is not just about innovation but also about delivering smarter, more connected care. Tools like telemedicine bridge distances and bring critical services to underserved communities. Wearable devices enable individuals to take charge of their health, and advanced analytics help clinicians make informed decisions in real-time. These technologies empower providers and patients alike, offering practical solutions to complex problems and unlocking possibilities for truly patient-centred care.

However, transformation requires more than technology: it also requires purpose-driven integration. Success in Digital Health means crafting solutions that seamlessly fit into clinical workflows and resonate with the people who use them. It means leveraging innovation to reduce provider burdens, engage patients meaningfully, and improve health outcomes. It means a commitment to usability, privacy, and trust, at both the patient and provider levels.

In this chapter, we explore the critical components for integrating Digital Health into Primary Care and offer a comprehensive view towards successful

DOI: 10.1201/9781003610519-8

adoption. From assessing readiness to addressing barriers and reimagining education, this chapter provides actionable insights for clinicians, administrators, and policymakers navigating this digital transformation journey.

ASSESSING PRACTICE READINESS FOR DIGITAL HEALTH INTEGRATION

Assessing practice readiness is a crucial first step in the successful integration of Digital Health solutions into Primary Care. Readiness encompasses a comprehensive evaluation of the healthcare ecosystem, considering the policy environment, technical capabilities, financial resources, and the competencies of both providers and patients. It also involves addressing regulatory and compliance issues to ensure secure and efficient implementation. This section explores these key factors that determine readiness and offers a roadmap for Primary Care practices to assess their capacity for digital transformation.

Policy and Leadership

Policy and leadership are key drivers of Digital Health readiness, especially in Primary Care. A supportive policy environment—through government mandates, institutional guidelines, and strategic plans—creates a foundation for innovation. For example, national policies that promote programs supporting digitalisation or health information exchange systems can accelerate the adoption of digital solutions in Primary Care by providing clear direction, allocating the appropriate funds, and reducing uncertainty for stakeholders.[2] Leadership also plays a crucial role in guiding Digital Health implementation. Leaders need to advocate for change, secure resources, address resistance, and align stakeholders with a shared vision for Digital Health adoption.[3]

An effective policy evaluation model is also essential. It should assess the impact of Digital Health initiatives across key areas, including strategy, governance, service delivery, workforce, Information Technology (IT) systems, and finances.[4] This approach helps ensure that digital tools align with institutional goals, address gaps, and support smooth integration into Primary Care workflows.

Infrastructure and Technological Capabilities

A key contextual factor is infrastructure, as it forms the backbone of any Digital Health initiative. Essential components include reliable internet access, electricity, adequate hardware (e.g., tablets, smartphones, and servers), and interoperable software systems. However, many Primary Care settings, particularly in rural or underserved areas, face significant infrastructure gaps, which similarly holds true for the patients in the populations that they serve.[4]

Closing these gaps requires strategic investments, such as expanding broadband access and providing grants for hardware acquisition. Countries and healthcare environments with more robust infrastructures have facilitated electronic health record (EHR) implementation and are more conducive to effective eHealth initiatives. It is important to consider both *proximal* infrastructure factors such as Primary Care practice capabilities and more *distal* factors such as country-wide internet availability and power. Addressing these technological needs is a prerequisite for achieving equitable and effective Digital Health integration.

Financial Readiness and Resource Allocation

The financial readiness of a Primary Care practice often determines the feasibility of adopting Digital Health solutions. Upfront costs, including software licensing and hardware procurement, can be a significant barrier, especially for smaller practices. Identifying and promoting sustainable financing models to support Digital Health development are key to support the corresponding financial burdens,[1] and financial arrangements should continue to adapt to accommodate new technologies that support coordination, interoperability, and regulation.[5]

Overcoming these barriers entails exploring cost-sharing models, public-private partnerships, and government subsidies. For instance, initiatives such as the US Health IT for Economic and Clinical Health (HITECH) Act have incentivised EHR adoption through financial assistance programs.[1] Additionally, for patients to fully take advantage of these new technologies, insurance schemes or pooled funding arrangements that include digital primary healthcare services are key. For example, when COVID-19 hit, financing arrangements were quickly adapted to enable necessary changes, such as extending benefit packages to include remote consultations.[5]

Digital Capabilities of Providers and Patients as Core Competencies

The digital literacy of both healthcare providers and patients is a critical determinant of readiness. Providers must be trained to use new tools effectively and to integrate them into their clinical workflows without compromising patient care.[6] Involving providers as end users in the development of digital systems may improve technology's usability, effectiveness, and, therefore, readiness from the Primary Care provider's point of view.[6]

Patients, in contrast, require accessible and user-friendly interfaces to engage with Digital Health solutions. Patients' digital capability readiness involves many aspects including users' knowledge and skills, their self-management of disease, their perceptions and mindset, their experience with health technology systems, and an understanding of the extent to which users feel supported by relatives, peers, and health professionals.[2] Strategies to enhance digital literacy, such as community workshops or patient education campaigns, are essential for fostering inclusivity and adoption.

Regulatory Compliance and Workflow Compatibility as Essential Alignments

Regulatory and compliance considerations are non-negotiable aspects of Digital Health readiness. Adhering to data protection laws, such as the Health Insurance Portability and Accountability Act (HIPAA) in the United States or the General Data Protection Regulation (GDPR) in the European Union, ensures the security and confidentiality of patient information. Data from primary healthcare is essential for informing national outbreak surveillance, understanding service pressures, fostering biomedical research, developing risk algorithms, and analysing inequalities to inform clinical and public health interventions (Pagliari, 2021).[7] Failure to comply with these regulations can lead to legal liabilities and the erosion of patient trust.

Workflow compatibility is another critical factor. Digital tools must align with existing clinical processes to avoid disruptions. Conducting workflow assessments and engaging frontline providers in the design and implementation process can help achieve this alignment. This should take place as early as possible in the process to achieve true co-creation. Digital systems' readiness depends on their flexibility to accommodate the varied needs of different primary healthcare practices, such as different workflows depending on staff and skills.

BOX 8.1   DIGITAL HEALTH EVALUATION/ASSESSMENT STRATEGIES/TOOLS

This textbox provides a variety of resources for assessing and/or guiding different readiness aspects for Digital Health implementation at the Primary Care level. It also includes broader implementation science assessment tools.

- **Digital Health and quality of care in PHC Evaluation Model:** A Digital Health evaluation model especially designed for PHC settings that assesses Structures (resources), Processes (activities), and Results (products, intermediate results, and impacts).[8]
- **Framework for Digital Health policy:** A Digital Health policy framework for a virtual Primary Care system that provides policy guiding principles for the following dimensions: Objectives;

Regulation/Governance; Delivery/Integration; Workforce; IT systems/Data sharing; and Financing/Reimbursement.[9]

- **The Primary Care (GP) Digital Services Operating Model** *(Securing Excellence in Primary Care (GP) Digital Services: The Primary Care (GP) Digital Services Operating Model 2021– 2023)*: A work that covers the key policies, standards, and operating procedures for the provision of high-quality general practice digital services. *Appendix D—Digital Primary Care maturity assurance tool indicators* in this document lists the set of indicators linked to a particular model's mandated requirement.
- **Digital First: GP readiness checklist:** A guide that provides support, resources, and a checklist for assessing primary healthcare practice readiness related to Digital Health capabilities.[10]
- **Hybrid Health Care Quality Assessment:** A self-assessment questionnaire (33 items) based on a Structure-Process-Outcome framework to evaluate the quality of hybrid care based on organisational, technological, process, and personal factors.[11]
- **eHealth methodology guide:** An online eHealth methodology guide to facilitate researchers and healthcare providers in selecting a suitable evaluation approach depending on the specific study phase.[12]
- **RE-AIM framework:** A well-known framework to evaluate science implementation that assesses key dimensions such as reach and effectiveness (individual level), adoption and implementation (staff, setting, system or policy levels), and maintenance (both the individual and staff/setting/system/ policy levels).[13]

IDENTIFYING AND OVERCOMING BARRIERS TO ADOPTION/ IMPLEMENTATION

Digital Health extends beyond designing new tools and developing modern methods in Primary Care delivery; it promotes and requires adopting these technologies and embedding them into existing healthcare systems. The key lies in the relationship between *technology development* and *practical implementation* to ensure intended improvements in service delivery. Technology development must be implementation-focused, and practical implementation should inform ongoing tool refinement to achieve optimal outcomes and sustainability.

The Consolidated Framework for Implementation Research (CFIR) offers a comprehensive lens to assess the implementation barriers that affect the adoption of Digital Health technologies in Primary Care.[14] CFIR addresses factors that span external and internal system dynamics, intervention and innovation domains, individual characteristics, and the implementation process itself.

System Barriers

The challenges of adopting Digital Health tools in Primary Care often begin well before tool development. Effective stakeholder engagement is critical to designing tools that meet the needs and goals of the healthcare system. This process must be guided by clear policies and regulations to ensure smooth development and implementation. Although international frameworks such as the Human-Organization-Technology Fit Framework provide valuable guidance, these models must be tailored to the specific context of each country and healthcare system. Developing coherent, context-specific policies is essential to avoid policy gaps and fragmentation that could hinder implementation.

One of the most significant system barriers is financial constraints, which can disrupt both implementation processes and long-term sustainability. Clear and sustainable funding models are essential. These should maximise the use of existing resources and enablers, including human resources, infrastructure, collaborations, prior initiatives, and lessons learned from earlier trials. It is important to realise that "resources" encompass more than just finances—they also include system innovations and flexibility, which can drive efficiency and enhance implementation efforts. Financial models must incorporate these broader elements to effectively support the practical adoption of Digital Health tools in Primary Care.

Technical Barriers

For Digital Health tools to be successfully implemented and integrated, their technical requirements must be clearly defined. Basic requirements include reliable internet access for both providers and patients, modern equipment, and IT support to address potential interoperability issues. More advanced needs include robust data exchange policies, privacy regulations, and effective software management tools.

Innovation plays a vital role in overcoming technical barriers and ensuring successful implementation. Disruptive innovation simplifies complex Digital Health tools, which makes them more accessible, affordable, and user-friendly for baseline users. Sustaining innovation focuses on enhancing existing working tools to make them more user-centred and adapting them to align with changes in Primary Care workflows and system structures. Together, these innovations address user and provider concerns while fostering adaptability to evolving system cultures and requirements.

Resistance to Change

Work-environmental factors often hinder the adoption and implementation of Digital Health technologies. At the core of these challenges is resistance to change, which involves both individual concerns and broader organisational norms. The technology acceptance model (TAM) better describes this resistance through two key concepts: perceived usefulness and perceived ease of use.[15] A Digital Health tool is more likely to succeed if users believe that it will enhance their daily practice and find it both simple and innovative to use. These perceptions significantly shape behaviours toward adopting and integrating new Digital Health tools into existing systems, helping to ease resistance to change. Technology adoption attitudes are influenced by individual factors, such as healthcare professionals' skills and experience, the internal work culture, and the policies of each Primary Care facility.

Resistance can be mitigated by involving both frontline healthcare professionals and end users early in the tool development and system design processes. Engaging these stakeholders ensures that the tools meet practical needs while fostering a sense of ownership and trust. Additionally, reviewing internal policies and workflows is crucial to enabling the seamless integration of new technologies without causing significant disruptions to daily operations.

Patient Acceptance and Engagement

Accepting change is a complex process influenced by both anticipated and lived experiences. Patients can either become strong advocates for Digital Health technologies in Primary Care or be the most difficult to convince. The theoretical framework of acceptability (TFA) identifies seven dimensions that influence patient acceptance of new interventions, such as Digital Health tools.[16] These dimensions include the perceived effectiveness of the tools, the patient's confidence in their ability to use them (self-efficacy), and the burden associated with learning and adapting to new systems.

The TFA highlights the importance of engaging patients both emotionally and cognitively when introducing new technologies. A patient's emotional attitude toward Digital Health tools plays a vital role in ensuring their acceptability and usability. This can be closely linked to the dimensions of ethicality, which reflects how well the tools align with patients' values, and intervention coherence, which relates to patients' understanding of how the tools work and their impact on care.

Another significant consideration is the opportunity cost involved in adopting Digital Health technologies. For instance, remote consultations may offer convenience, but they could also reduce face-to-face interactions with healthcare providers or disrupt the continuity of care with the same practitioner. Addressing these concerns requires a thorough assessment of all dimensions at every stage of the process.

It is essential to consider patient acceptability proactively during tool design to ensure that their needs are met—adaptively during implementation to respond to feedback, and retrospectively for monitoring and evaluation. This approach ensures continuous improvement and promotes the successful integration of Digital Health technologies into Primary Care systems.

Main Enablers

The nonadoption, abandonment, scale-up, spread, and sustainability (NASSS) framework for health and care technologies shows that the wider institutional, policy, and sociocultural contexts have often been identified as key factors in the failure of an organisation to move from a demonstration project to a mainstreamed service that was transferable and sustainable (Figure 8.1).[17] Digital Health technologies co-created or supported by professional bodies and patient groups are more likely to be successfully implemented and respond to the needs of users over time.

Training and Skills Development

The successful integration and implementation of Digital Health technologies in Primary Care depends not only on the quality and functionality of the tools but also on the readiness and skills of the workforce to incorporate them seamlessly into daily practice. A well-trained healthcare professional who confidently and effectively uses digital tools enhances patient trust and satisfaction while also reducing the cognitive and operational burden of adapting to new systems. Moreover, fostering a culture of continuous skill development promotes lifelong learning and adaptability, which are crucial as Digital Health technologies continue to evolve. This approach ensures that healthcare providers can maximise the potential of these innovations in both Primary Care and across the broader healthcare system.

PRIMARY HEALTHCARE EDUCATION AND TRAINING

Healthcare providers require continuous, targeted education and training to effectively implement and utilise Digital Health in Primary Care. This need spans the entire spectrum of medical education, from undergraduate curricula to vocational training and continuing professional development (CPD).

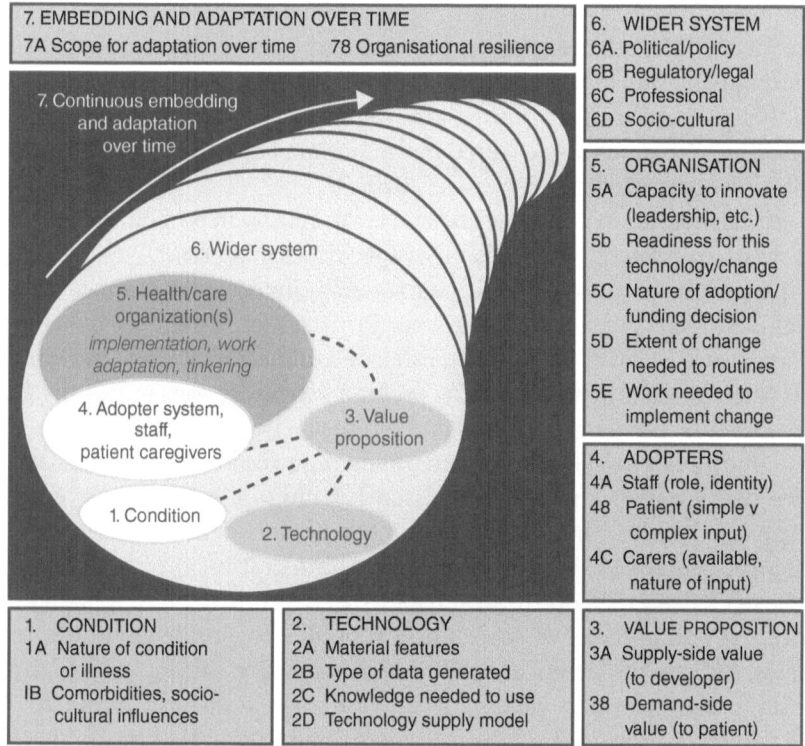

FIGURE 8.1 The NASSS framework for considering influences on the adoption, nonadoption, abandonment, spread, scale-up, and sustainability of patient-facing health and care technologies. *Source:* Greenhalgh T, Wherton J, Papoutsi C, Lynch J, Hughes G, A'Court C, Hinder S, Fahy N, Procter R, Shaw S Beyond Adoption: A New Framework for Theorizing and Evaluating Nonadoption, Abandonment, and Challenges to the Scale-Up, Spread, and Sustainability of Health and Care Technologies. *J Med Internet Res* 2017;19(11):e367 URL: https://www.jmir.org/2017/11/e367 https://doi.org/10.2196/jmir.8775 ©Trisha Greenhalgh, Joseph Wherton, Chrysanthi Papoutsi, Jennifer Lynch, Gemma Hughes, Christine A'Court, Susan Hinder, Nick Fahy, Rob Procter, Sara Shaw. Originally published in the *Journal of Medical Internet Research* (http://www.jmir.org), 01.11.2017.

CPD involves various educational activities that enable healthcare providers to keep their skills, knowledge, and relationships up to date in an ever-evolving field, aligning with new trends and practices.[18] This section explores the key areas of Digital Health education: assessing training needs, curriculum integration, training modalities, digital literacy for healthcare professionals, and sustained development programs.

The need for education and training in the field of Digital Health is widely acknowledged. In a large study across the eight university hospitals of the Netherlands, it was found that educational and implementation strategies, including practical skills training, are needed to help the upscaling of tele-monitoring.[19] This was also covered in the National eHealth vision developed by the University Medical Centers in 2020.

A crucial first step in designing Digital Health education programs is conduct-ing a needs assessment, which identifies specific learning objectives relevant to practitioners' everyday needs.[20] A scoping review by Jimenez et al. outlined the core Digital Health competencies necessary for Primary Care providers and empha-sised areas such as data management, patient communication, and telemedicine. Needs assessments help tailor training programs to bridge gaps in existing skills and prepare practitioners for current and future practice demands.[21]

Integrating Digital Health into curricula requires a strong foundation in faculty development and contextualised learning objectives. This ensures that subjects like health informatics and telemedicine are effectively taught. Challenges remain in determining optimal integration timing and depth, as little evidence exists on the best balance between instruction quality and quantity. A comprehensive curriculum should incorporate emerging tech-nologies, address the practical needs of Primary Care, and account for adult learning preferences and varying levels of digital literacy. A recent review noted that few medical schools have implemented Digital Health components in their programs, despite the growing role of these technologies in health-care—this is a missed opportunity for preparing future-ready practitioners.[22] An illustrative statement by Bhopal is, "the physicians of tomorrow are taught by the teachers of today using the curriculum of the past".[23]

Regarding continuous learning, CPD programs are essential for keep-ing Primary Care professionals up to date with Digital Health innovations. An opinion paper by Houwink et al. described what is required regarding Digital Health education for Primary Care professionals and trainees; fur-thermore, suggestions were provided on how Digital Health education could be provided.[24] The authors identified four key Digital Health education areas in Primary Care: understanding evidence-based Digital Health appli-cations, essential digital competencies for providers and patients, impacts of Digital Health on provider-patient relationships, and data management skills. Despite these recommendations, a 2023 study noted that the literature on practical training approaches and competencies remains limited, which highlights the need for interdisciplinary and public health-focused training.[25] The DigiCanTrain project provides further insights by mapping current CPD offerings across 25 EU countries, revealing significant variations in policy, training organisation, and funding, with a call for a systematic, equitable approach to digital skills training across Europe.[26]

Several training modalities are suggested for Digital Health education including blended learning, e-learning, and real-life practice simulations. Hands-on experience is crucial, as emphasised by Alhur et al., who advocate integrating Digital Health into clinical practice.[27] Frameworks such as CanMEDS and Kern's conceptual model provide structured approaches for setting learning goals and implementing Digital Health education.[24] Guided by a systematic needs assessment and collaboration with key stakeholders, the program aims to meet accreditation standards and is designed to be accessible to geographically dispersed providers, including those in rural and remote areas. The online CPD was well received, although evidence on its effectiveness is lacking (Figure 8.2).

The main objective of Digital Health training and education is for Primary Care providers to achieve a minimum level of digital literacy. On the one

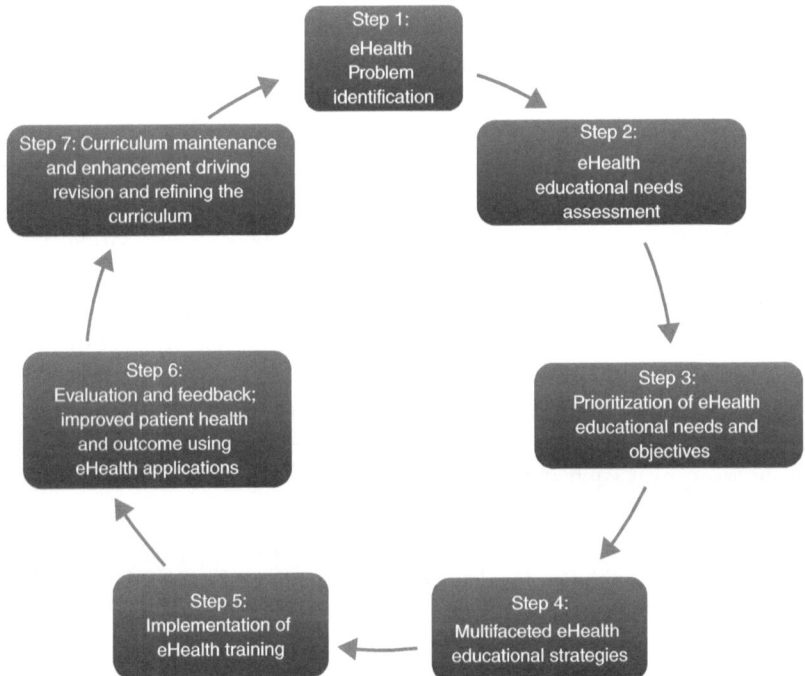

FIGURE 8.2 Conceptual model for the development, evaluation, and maintenance of a Digital Health education program. *Source:* Houwink EJF, Kasteleyn MJ, Alpay L, et al. SERIES: eHealth in primary care. Part 3: eHealth education in primary care. *Eur J Gen Pract.* 2020 Dec;26(1): 108–118. https://doi.org/10.1080/13814788.2020.1797675. © 2020 The Author(s). Published by Informa UK Limited, trading as Taylor & Francis Group.

hand, several initiatives highlight best practices in Digital Health education, which directly contribute to this goal. The SaNuRN project in France offers comprehensive Digital Health training for medical and paramedical students, leveraging the French National Referential on Digital Health (FNRDH).[28] The program includes competency-based evaluations, real-world telemedicine scenarios, and interactive video capsules that aim to train a significant portion of France's healthcare students by 2027. Another example is the Catalog and Index of Digital Health Teaching Resources (CIDHR), a multilingual semantic search engine that provides a centralised, accessible repository of high-quality Digital Health resources.[29] CIDHR enhances Digital Health literacy and supports knowledge sharing at various training levels.

On the other hand, Digital Health literacy will enable Primary Care practitioners to extend their role as Digital Health *mentors* for their patients. They are uniquely positioned to guide patients in adopting and effectively using Digital Health tools, bridging the gap between technology and patient-centred care. This requires them to balance technical proficiency with strong teaching and mentoring capabilities. Next to having a solid understanding of functionalities and limitations of tools, they need communication and mentoring skills that enable providers to translate this knowledge into meaningful guidance. Teaching patients—many of whom may be unfamiliar or uncomfortable with technology—requires a tailored approach.[24] Providers must assess the patient's digital literacy, address their concerns with empathy, and break down complex instructions into manageable steps. Moreover, fostering a sense of trust and empowerment is essential, especially for patients who may feel overwhelmed by the dual challenges of managing a chronic condition and adopting a new digital tool.

Finally, effective integration of Digital Health training within medical curricula requires multidisciplinary collaboration and practical, hands-on learning. Programs such as Stanford's Biodesign initiative, which bridges the gaps among medicine, engineering, and business, illustrate the benefits of partnerships across disciplines to equip future healthcare providers with the skills needed to use Digital Health tools effectively and safely.[22]

REFERENCES

1. WHO. *Global strategy on digital health 2020–2025*. Geneva: World Health Organization; 2021. Licence: CC BY-NC-SA 3.0 IGO. Accessed 2024 Nov 22. Available from: https://iris.who.int/bitstream/handle/10665/344249/9789240020924-eng.pdf.
2. Kayser L, Rossen S, Karnoe A, et al. Development of the multidimensional readiness and enablement index for health technology (READHY) tool to measure individuals' health technology readiness: initial testing in a cancer rehabilitation setting. *J Med Internet Res*. 2019;21(2):e10377. https://doi.org/10.2196/10377.
3. Erku D, Khatri R, Endalamaw A, et al. Digital health interventions to improve access to and quality of primary health care services: a scoping review. *Int J Environ Res Public Health*. 2023;20:6854. https://doi.org/10.3390/ijerph20196854.

4. Silva ÍDS, Silva CRDV, Martiniano CS, et al. Digital health and quality of care in primary health care: an evaluation model. *Front Public Health.* 2022;12:1443862. https://doi.org/10.3389/fpubh.2024.144386.

5. Hanson K, Brikci N, Erlangga D, et al. The Lancet global health commission on financing primary health care: putting people at the centre. *The Lancet Glob Health.* 2022;10(5):e715–72.

6. Alotaibi N, Brown Wilson C, Traynor M, et al. Enhancing digital readiness and capability in healthcare: a systematic review of interventions, barriers, and facilitators. *Preprint (Version 1) Res Sq.* 2024 Aug 28. https://doi.org/10.21203/rs.3.rs-4816097/v1.

7. Pagliari C. Digital health and primary care: past, pandemic and prospects. *J Glob Health.* 2021 Jul 2;11:01005. https://doi.org/10.7189/jogh.11.01005.

8. Silva ÍDS, Silva CRDV, Martiniano CS, Araújo AJD, Figueirêdo RCD, Lapão LV, Moioli RC, Brito EWG and Uchôa SadC. Digital health and quality of care in Primary Health Care: An evaluation model. *Front Public Health* 2024;12:1443862. https://doi.org/10.3389/fpubh.2024.1443862.

9. Srivastava D, Van Kessel R, Delgrange M, Cherla A, Sood H, Mossialos E. A framework for digital health policy: Insights from virtual primary care systems across five nations. *PLOS Digit Health* 2023;2(11): e0000382. https://doi.org/10.1371/journal.pdig.0000382.

10. NHS, Digital First, *Support and Resource Guide V2.* South East Region GP Practices; 2024.

11. Tossaint-Schoenmakers R, Kasteleyn MJ, Rauwerdink A, Chavannes N, Willems S, Talboom-Kamp EPWA. Development of a quality management model and self-assessment questionnaire for hybrid health care: Concept mapping study. *JMIR Form Res.* 2022 Jul 7;6(7):e38683. https://doi.org/10.2196/38683.

12. Bonten TN, Rauwerdink A, Wyatt JC, Kasteleyn MJ, Witkamp L, Riper H, van Gemert-Pijnen LJ, Cresswell K, Sheikh A, Schijven MP, Chavannes NH, EHealth Evaluation Research Group. Online guide for electronic health evaluation approaches: Systematic scoping review and concept mapping study. *J Med Internet Res* 2020;22(8):e17774. https://doi.org/10.2196/17774.

13. Holtrop JS, Estabrooks PA, Gaglio B, et al. Understanding and applying the RE-AIM framework: Clarifications and resources. *J Clin Trans Sci* 2021;5(1):e126. https://doi.org/10.1017/cts.2021.789.

14. Damschroder LJ, Reardon CM, Widerquist, MAO, et al. The updated consolidated framework for implementation research based on user feedback. *Implement Sci.* 2022;17:75. https://doi.org/10.1186/s13012-022-01245-0.

15. Kalayou MH, Endehabtu BF, Tilahun B. The applicability of the modified technology acceptance model (TAM) on the sustainable adoption of eHealth systems in resource-limited settings. *J Multidiscip Healthc.* 2020 Dec 3;13:1827–37. https://doi.org/10.2147/JMDH.S284973.

16. Sekhon M, Cartwright M, Francis JJ, et al. Acceptability of healthcare interventions: an overview of reviews and development of a theoretical framework. *BMC Health Serv Res.* 2017;17:88. https://doi.org/10.1186/s12913-017-2031-8.

17. Greenhalgh T, Wherton J, Papoutsi C, et al. Beyond adoption: a new framework for theorizing and evaluating nonadoption, abandonment, and challenges to the scale-up, spread, and sustainability of health and care technologies. *J Med Internet Res.* 2017;19(11):e367. https://www.jmir.org/2017/11/e367; https://doi.org/10.2196/jmir.8775.

18. Curran V, Hollett A, Peddle E. Training for virtual care: what do the experts think? *Digit Health.* 2023;9. https://doi.org/10.1177/20552076231179028.

19. Gijsbers HJH, Kleiss J, Nurmohamed SA, et al. Upscaling telemonitoring in Dutch university medical centres: a baseline measurement. *Int J Med Inform.* 2023;175:105085. https://doi.org/10.1016/j.ijmedinf.2023.105085.

20. Al-Ismail MS, Naseralallah LM, Hussain TA, et al. Learning needs assessments in continuing professional development: a scoping review. *Med Teach*. 2023 Feb;45(2):203–11. https://doi.org/10.1080/0142159X.2022.2126756. Epub 2022 Sep 30.

21. Jimenez G, Spinazze P, Matchar D, et al. Digital health competencies for primary healthcare professionals: a scoping review. *Int J Med Inform*. 2020;143:104260. https://doi.org/10.1016/j.ijmedinf.2020.104260.

22. Boillat T, Otaki F, Baghestani A, et al. A landscape analysis of digital health technology in medical schools: preparing students for the future of health care. *BMC Med Educ*. 2024;24:1011. https://doi.org/10.1186/s12909-024-06006-9.

23. Bhopal A. Attitude and the 21st century doctor. *Lancet Glob Health*. 2015;3(3):e126–7.

24. Houwink EJF, Kasteleyn MJ, Alpay L, et al. SERIES: eHealth in primary care. Part 3: eHealth education in primary care. *Eur J Gen Pract*. 2020 Dec;26(1):108–18. https://doi.org/10.1080/13814788.2020.1797675.

25. Ramachandran S, Chang HJ, Worthington C, et al. Digital competencies and training approaches to enhance the capacity of practitioners to support the digital transformation of public health: rapid review of current recommendations. *JMIR Public Health Surveill*. 2024 Sep 9;10:e52798. https://doi.org/10.2196/52798.

26. Kaihlanen AM, Virtanen L, Kainiemi E, et al. Continuing education in digital skills for healthcare professionals—mapping of the current situation in EU member states. *Int J Health Policy Manag*. 2024;13:8309. https://doi.org/10.34172/ijhpm.8309. Epub 2024 Jun 24.

27. Alhur AA. Integrating digital health into medical curricula: a review of current practices and future directions. *Int J Biosci*. 2023 Dec;23(6):34–43.

28. Grosjean J, Dufour F, Benis A, et al. Digital health education for the future: the SaNuRN (Santé Numérique Rouen-Nice) consortium's journey. *JMIR Med Educ*. 2024 Apr 30;10:e53997. https://doi.org/10.2196/53997.

29. Grosjean J, Benis A, Dufour JC, et al. Sharing digital health educational resources in a one-stop shop portal: tutorial on the catalog and index of digital health teaching resources (CIDHR) semantic search engine. *JMIR Med Educ*. 2024 Mar 4;10:e48393. https://doi.org/10.2196/48393.

CHAPTER 9

Digital Health Sustainability and Systems Thinking Approaches

Nick Guldemond, Melita Sogomonjan, and Mariam Beridze

DIGITAL HEALTH SUSTAINABILITY IN THE CONTEXT OF SYSTEMS THINKING APPROACHES

Digital Health sustainability and related Systems Thinking approaches have multiple dimensions and various levels—which are essential for making the development, implementation, up-scaling and consolidation of accessible, good quality and person-centred services.[1] Digital Health services, including those provided from a Primary Care perspective, are intrinsically dependent on the conditions determined by health system policies. In other words, it is unlikely that Digital Health initiatives in Primary Care will be successful if the various health system requirements (i.e., legal-regulatory, funding and reimbursement, integration and interoperability, workforce training and development, and equity) are not appropriately addressed and aligned. Health Systems Thinking approaches are therefore essential for sustainable development and the implementation and upscaling of Primary Care-based Digital Health services.[2]

Health systems worldwide are facing challenges due to longstanding fragmentation in services, technology, governance and finances. The demand for more complex care is increasing because of an aging population and a rising number of people with chronic conditions. This is creating an unmanageable burden on health systems. In addition to the gradual increase in demographic

DOI: 10.1201/9781003610519-9

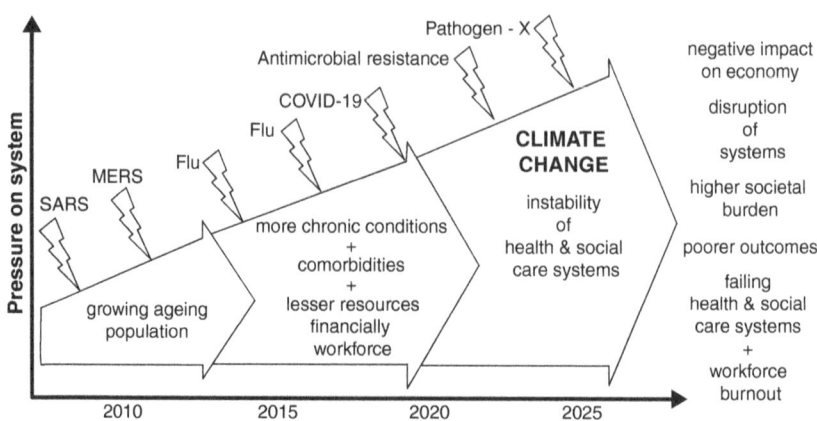

FIGURE 9.1 The challenges of health systems. The prevalent challenges faced by modern health systems, include ageing populations, the increasing burden of chronic diseases and constraints on human and financial resources. At the same time, emerging public health threats—such as climate change—are exacerbating system instability, with widespread consequences for both society and the economy as a whole.

pressure, the COVID-19 pandemic revealed the weaknesses of health and social care systems in addressing sudden health crises. Most healthcare systems are not considered resilient to shocks like infectious outbreaks or other societal health threats such as antimicrobial resistance and climate change (Figure 9.1).[3]

Accordingly, health system sustainability has become a broader concept in recent years and now goes beyond the traditional focus on human and financial resources. The stark consequences of climate change and the COVID-19 pandemic showed the inherent interconnectedness of human health and care services, animal health and environmental health—a concept known as 'One Health' (Figure 9.2). One Health is a collaborative, multisectoral and transdisciplinary approach. It aims to achieve optimal health outcomes and recognise the interconnection among people, animals, plants and their shared environment while working at the local, regional, national and global levels (Figure 9.2).[4]

From a holistic systems point of view, human health, animal health and environmental health co-exist within our planet and are influenced by global factors such as climate, natural disasters, resources and energy. Viewing the healthcare system as a whole has implications for all policies (rather than focusing on individual components and sectors) and helps in identifying how different parts of the system affect one another. The socio-economic, political, and cultural contexts play critical roles in shaping transformation towards more sustainable health systems.

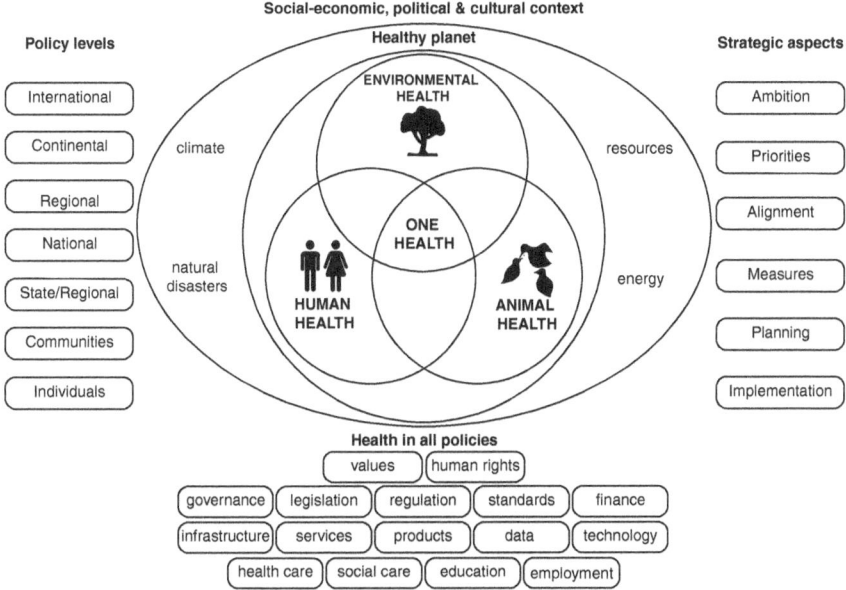

FIGURE 9.2 The One Health Approach, a holistic framework for health

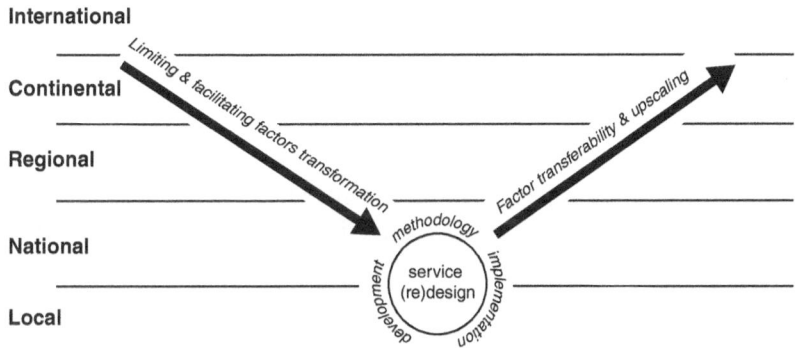

FIGURE 9.3 A policy multi-level approach to implementation and upscaling system transformation.

Furthermore, implementing system transformations that include a digital component require a comprehensive strategy that encompasses the entire health system: from a global policy level to an operational local level, and vice versa (Figure 9.3).[5] Effective implementation of the One Health vision involves setting ambitions and priorities, ensuring the alignment of goals and adopting strategic measures and planning.

This vision applies to the development, implementation and upscaling of digital innovation and to the consolidation of existing digitally enabled services where Primary Care, secondary care, community services, prevention and patient self-management are smoothly integrated and work together in an effective way to deliver care.

International collaboration between regional ecosystems can speed the implementation and expansion of successful practices by sharing knowledge and exchanging experiences. Figure 9.3 illustrates a multi-level approach to implementing and upscaling initiatives within a healthcare or public health context. It emphasises the interplay between different levels, from international to local, and the factors that influence success at each stage. However, resources for health systems are finite and require creative and effective uses. This chapter addresses a system-wide approach to achieve Digital Health sustainability. Furthermore, it demonstrates the opportunities for improvement that can potentially drive reforms of health systems that improve their accessibility, effectiveness, equity and sustainability.

VALUES AND PRINCIPLES OF PERSON-CENTRED DIGITAL HEALTH IN PRIMARY CARE

Every health system uses certain values and guiding principles by which medical practice, health and social services are organised.[6] Typically, these consist of more general and specific values, including the following:

- **Availability:** ensuring that services and essential health commodities are *accessible* and consistently *available* to those who need them.
- **Accessibility**: ensuring that services are affordable and accessible for all individuals and communities, including those in remote or underserved areas.
- **Acceptability:** health services delivered in a manner that is respectful of individuals' culture, gender, age and other social and personal characteristics.
- **Appropriateness:** delivery of services that are evidence-based and of high quality and that meet the needs of the population being served.
- **Accountability:** ensuring that health systems are transparent, responsive and responsible.
- **People at the centre:** to serve and benefit people and empower them to pursue their aspirations, without infringing their security or fundamental rights.
- **Solidarity and inclusion:** inclusion and promotion of patients' and citizens' rights, ensuring that Digital Health solutions are accessible to all, regardless of their socio-economic status, location or background.

- **Freedom of choice:** patients and citizens should be empowered to make their own informed choices.
- **Participation**: engagement and democratic processes through trustworthy, diverse and multilingual environments.
- **Safety and security**: safe, secure and privacy-protective technologies, products and services that protect patient data through robust privacy and security measures to ensure confidentiality and trust.
- **Sustainability**: digital and green transitions are closely linked; although digital technologies offer many solutions for climate change, we must acknowledge that digitalisation increases energy consumption and resources to bring innovations for consumption.

DIGITAL HEALTH SUSTAINABILITY

Digital Health sustainability refers to the practice of developing, implementing and upscaling Digital Health solutions in a way that ensures that they are environmentally, economically and socially sustainable for a long period of time. Additionally, sustainable Digital Health must be inherently adaptable to evolving needs, technological advancements and shifting societal contexts. Accordingly, a sustainable Digital Health strategy has to strike a delicate balance that ensures long-term plans with clear objectives, strategic actions and planning and that allows flexibility in terms of governance structures so that it can quickly respond to new information, challenges and opportunities. This should facilitate a culture of continuous learning and improvement while encouraging feedback and innovation to refine Digital Health solutions.[7]

During the COVID-19 pandemic, many healthcare systems demonstrated this duality by swiftly expanding telehealth services to meet the urgent needs of patients while maintaining a long-term vision for integrating Digital Health into routine care. By combining a consistent, long-term plan with the flexibility to adapt, a sustainable Digital Health strategy can effectively address both current and future healthcare challenges.[8]

As discussed in the previous chapter, implementing digitally enabled person-centred care models requires a comprehensive implementation strategy that encompasses the entire health system with its various levels as presented in Figure 9.3. The implication is that successful Digital Health implementation and system-wide changes are inherently linked and should be part of an overall multi-dimensional and multi-level strategy.[9]

FINANCIAL DIGITAL HEALTH SUSTAINABILITY

Financial sustainability in Digital Health is an interdependent, multifaceted challenge that spans different phases of development, implementation, actual use and upscaling solutions.[10]

- **Development phase:** Initial investments are needed to secure funding for research and development. This usually comes from government grants, private investors or public-private partnerships. Cost-benefit analyses are needed to ensure that the proposed Digital Health solution is financially viable and offers a good return on investment.[11]
- **Implementation phase:** For implementation, it is necessary to allocate sufficient budget for the deployment of Digital Health solutions, including infrastructure, training and support systems. Conducting pilot programs can help test the usability, feasibility, clinical effectiveness and cost-effectiveness of the solution before full-scale implementation.
- **Use phase:** The total cost of ownership (TCO) should be considered when the eventual use of the Digital Health solution is imminent. This is essential for evaluating the financial viability and overall value of a Digital Health investment. The TCO in the context of Digital Health solutions encompasses all expenses associated with acquiring, deploying and maintaining these technologies throughout their lifecycle. Acquisition costs comprise hardware, software and infrastructure. Deployment costs are associated with configuring the technology, including installation, setup and initial support, integrating Digital Health solutions into existing healthcare systems and workflows, training staff, changing management and earmarking ongoing operational costs such as maintenance, updates and support services. It is also important to consider the 'hidden costs'. These are costs associated with system downtime, including lost productivity, patient dissatisfaction and potential revenue loss, and costs related to data breaches (i.e., fines, legal fees and reputational damage).[12]
- **Upscaling phase:** It is important to confirm that the Digital Health solution can be scaled up efficiently without significant additional costs while leveraging economies of scale to reduce per-unit costs as the solution is adopted by more users or institutions.[13]

By addressing these aspects at each phase, Digital Health solutions can achieve financial sustainability to ensure that they remain viable and beneficial in the long term. A sustainable Digital Health business model cannot exist without a thorough understanding and management of the TCO. This ensures financial viability, enables long-term planning and strengthens the value proposition of a Primary Care organisation (for both patients and the payors). Meanwhile, it is essential to secure continuous funding through grants, investments and/or partnerships to support the maintenance, improvement and expansion of the solution.

Regulatory provisions and financial incentives play a significant role in the implementation of a digitally enabled health ecosystem. Aligned regulations can make it easier to adopt interoperability standards, share data and use digital service platforms. Financial incentives can also motivate provider organisations to adopt digitally enabled care through pay-for-performance and value-based payment models.[14]

LEGAL AND REGULATORY REQUIREMENTS FOR DIGITAL HEALTH SUSTAINABILITY

Legal and regulatory requirements are a prerequisite for ensuring the sustainability of Digital Health. Legal frameworks for processing health data, such as the General Data Protection Regulation (GDPR) in Europe, the Health Insurance Portability and Accountability Act (HIPAA) in the United States and many other national regulations worldwide, are essential not only for the protection of health data but also for their functional and effective use. Legal and regulatory provisions should aim to:

- Promote interoperability standards to ensure that Digital Health systems can communicate and share data seamlessly;
- Ensure that Digital Health solutions are safe and effective, provide clinical value and offer guidance on regulatory approval before they can be marketed and used in practice;
- Safeguard intellectual assets via patents, copyrights and trademarks to facilitate innovation and enable inventors to receive a return on their efforts; and
- Provide guidance on liability and risk management while addressing the potential legal issues related to the use of Digital Health innovations.

The discussions around the development of integrated health systems and the One Health vision have intensified in the context of emerging pandemics and climate change. These challenges highlight the importance of data sharing to facilitate decision making and the prevention of emerging public health threats in order to anticipate emergencies and improve crisis responses.[15] The Food and Agriculture Organization of the United Nations has outlined the areas where appropriate legislation should be implemented. Still, inconsistencies persist among national, European Union (EU) and international legislation concerning the protection of environmental health including animal health, food safety and quality and antimicrobial resistance.[16] The implementation and enforcement of a unified sustainable One Health approach remains difficult due to the inadequate coordination and integration of animal-human-environmental sectors across countries. In addition to technical challenges, inconsistent and fragmented regulations address sector-specific technical, financial and organisational issues.[17] For example, a lack of guidelines regarding antibiotic prescriptions and related healthcare data collection and monitoring in Primary Care can lead to the overuse or misuse of antibiotics that eventually results in antimicrobial resistance.[18] Antimicrobial resistance is a huge public health threat (Figure 9.1) that was listed among the top ten threats to global health in 2019.[19] Nevertheless, the current public health laws do not adequately address public health threats in a comprehensive, aligned way: antimicrobial resistance lacks proper measures to prevent inadequate prescribing through digital monitoring.

The lack of utilisation of cross-sectoral data also leads to inappropriate and poor management of public health threats in the primary health care (PHC) system. The legal opacity and uncertainties are increasing the complexity of integrating innovation into healthcare and cross-sectoral communication. Therefore, an adequate infrastructure to support integrated health systems and the modernisation of current regulatory pathways are essential for the success of a data-driven One Health approach.[20] The recently approved EU Artificial Intelligence Act has the potential to harmonise legislation concerning data sharing across sectors and accelerate the implementation of integrated health systems, both at the local and regional (EU) levels. It is highly expected that AI-generated tools will increase the accuracy of documentation, diagnosis, treatment, management of care and follow-up visits.[21]

In general, health data processing must comply with the following basic legal principles:[22]

- First, health data must be processed lawfully and fairly, and transparent free, specific, informed and unambiguous consent must be given. In the context of the EU's GDPR, healthcare providers are allowed to share health data for primary and secondary uses with the informed consent of the patient or their legal representative. To accelerate the implementation of integrated health systems and person-centred digitally enabled health and social care, tech-friendly laws have been adopted to allow health data sharing on the basis of opt-out consent. This implies that the processing of health data is given by default through secure information systems.
- Second, the processing of health data must be accurate and minimal (i.e., only the essential personal data are collected and analysed) and kept confidential. Data should be used for the original purpose or adjusted with informed consent and removed if they are not necessary or if consent is withdrawn. Having an opportunity to exercise control over the access, accuracy and integrity of health data has been acknowledged as a basic human right.

Although the availability of accurate and complete healthcare data is essential for the functioning of integrated health systems and digitally enabled care, it has been agreed that opt-out consent will remain voluntarily for Member States to implement.[23] Member States have the right to introduce limitations and justified exceptions regarding the processing of health, genetic and biometric data.[24]

The national laws on data protection may vary regardless of EU and international health policies and regulations. Currently, data protection laws are focused on preventing unauthorised access and maintaining patient confidentiality and privacy. The need to comply with national data protection laws and regulations may still impede the implementation of integrated health systems and digitally enabled health and social care in primary and cross-border care. Concomitantly, the legal framework for data protection must be re-evaluated in the context of the emerging benefits that integrated health systems provide to maintain the sustainability of the PHC system. To accelerate the practices of cross-border telehealth services in the EU, the initial proposal for the European Health Data Space (EHDS) regulation included provisions stipulating the harmonisation of legal requirements. Article 8 of the proposal included "Whether a Member State accepts the provision of telemedicine services, it shall, under the same conditions, accept the provision of the services of the same type by healthcare providers located in other Member States."[25] Nevertheless, this provision was removed by the European Council during the ongoing legislative process.[26] The legislation and regulations in the United States (US), United Kingdom (UK) and many other countries largely have the same provisions. Data sharing to facilitate integrated health systems and person-centred digitally enabled care is possible in many jurisdictions as long as informed consent is provided and compliance with legal and regulatory requirements is met.

Currently, access to cross-border telehealth services and the subsequent reimbursement costs remain largely fragmented and depend on the eligibility criteria and regulatory and administrative formalities of each country.[27] The fragmentation and variability in reimbursement for cross-border telehealth services are not unique to the EU. Other continents also face similar challenges. In many EU countries and in the UK and Australia, the laws governing the provision of healthcare apply to telehealth.[28] In the US, however, the delivery of telehealth services is regulated at the state level. This can create challenges, as legal inconsistencies and fragmentation may reduce the ability to fully address the complex and evolving changes in contemporary healthcare delivery models.[26]

Effective integrated health systems have the potential to improve the sustainability of PHC systems and quality of life. But so far, investments in the digitalisation of healthcare have been oriented to improve efficiency in management and the organisation of the healthcare system, establishing control, coordination and financing mechanisms. Less attention has been devoted to the practical use of Digital Health technology, including investments in the digitalisation of multiple sectors to communicate and work together for the purposes of achieving better public health outcomes.[29] Considering the need for an alignment of the different dimensions and sectors, a comprehensive legal framework is required to facilitate sustainable, digitally enabled Primary Care. This framework should encompass regulations for inter-sectoral collaboration and control and coordination mechanisms to support effective implementation.[30]

POLICY STRATEGY AND PLANNING TO ACHIEVE DIGITAL HEALTH SUSTAINABILITY

As presented in the introduction to this chapter, health systems are faced with multiple challenges, which should be considered in the current context of economic volatility, technological disruption, geopolitical tensions and political instability. These developments all cast potential negative ripple effects on health systems and service continuity. Securing health systems performance and continuity in volatile times requires a comprehensive policy strategy and planning approach that should anticipate both slowly developing trends (i.e., a rising demand for healthcare services and a gradual reduction of resources) and sudden high-impact incidents (i.e., health emergencies).

Political instability and a rapidly changing healthcare context make long-term planning more challenging. As a result, leaders often react and make decisions based on immediate pressures rather than on a long-term vision or strategy. Effective strategic planning often requires opportunistic responses to health and economic issues and rapidly evolving technological developments. Although the potential benefits of digitalisation and healthcare innovation are captivating, the focus on the core elements of strategic planning remain more crucial than ever.

Strategic planning starts with a 'crystal clear' mission definition, which should go beyond crafting vision statements. Strategic planning is a continuous process and involves informed choices about which scenarios to pursue and which to ignore. These decisions have impacts on resource allocation, capacity building, technology investments and funding strategies. This requires policymakers to precisely articulate their short- and long-term organisational strategy, related objectives, proposed actions to achieve these objectives, the roles and responsibilities of the people executing them, realistic planning and a budget. Strategic planning also includes contingency plans to address critical events and dependencies that could potentially place health systems at risk, such as disrupted operational productivity, threats to the integrity of critical digital infrastructure and the loss or breach of sensitive data (e.g., cyberattacks).

The Ambrose Model of Change for managing complex change (Figure 9.4)[31] provides a holistic framework for managing change within organisations that can be applied to Digital Health sustainability. This model has the following steps:

- Define a vision for a sustainable Digital Health region-oriented ecosystem, with the involvement of all relevant providers and actors, that is focused on the improvement of patient outcomes, cost reduction and increased accessibility.
- Build capacity and train professionals through continuous education and post-graduate programs to keep them updated with the latest Digital Health technologies and practices.
- Implement Digital Health policies that provide financial incentives for providers who adopt and effectively use Digital Health solutions.
- Allocate funding and resources to support the development and maintenance of Digital Health infrastructure, including broadband connectivity and secure data storage.
- Create a comprehensive action plan that includes specific goals, strategies and timelines for implementing Digital Health initiatives. Regularly review and update the plan to adapt to changing needs and circumstances.

The Ambrose Model of Change posits that the presence or absence of each element can significantly impact the outcome of a change initiative. When all elements are present, the effect is likely to be successful. However, the

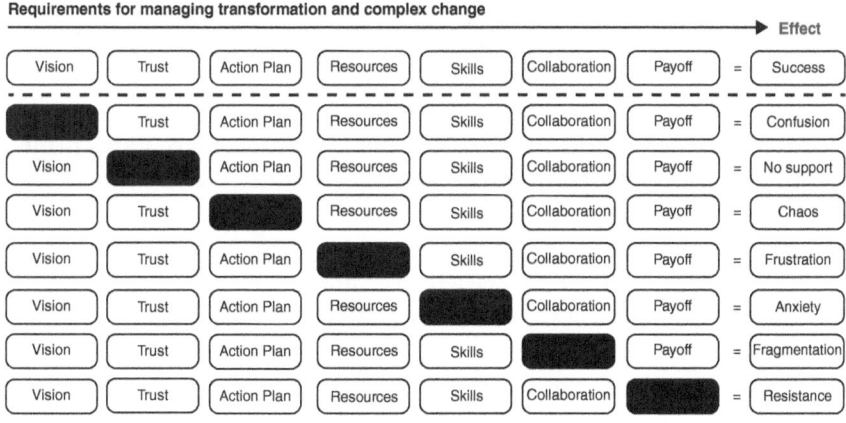

FIGURE 9.4 The Ambrose model for managing complex change.

absence of any one element can lead to negative outcomes. This approach should ensure that health policies are aligned with broader societal goals, such as universal health coverage and health equity.

Translating the values and principles described above into a policy strategy within the context of an appropriate legal and regulatory framework for Digital Health involves several steps, as follows:

- Engagement with stakeholders, including healthcare providers, patients, policymakers and technology developers, to gather input and ensure that the policy framework addresses their needs and concerns.
- Evaluation of existing policies and legal and regulatory frameworks to assess whether they not only are adequate and aligned with the needs and concerns of the stakeholders but also meet the requirements that commonly apply to Digital Health (e.g., data protection laws, medical device regulations and telemedicine guidelines).
- Integration of legal and regulatory requirements into the design and development of Digital Health solutions from the outset to ensure that adoption and compliance are built into the provision of services.[32]
- Conduction of a risk assessment to identify the potential legal and regulatory challenges to mitigate these risks in the development and execution of policy strategies.

Collaborative action is needed that unites researchers, professionals, patients and providers. Involving patients and all relevant stakeholders through co-creation approaches should ensure the development of concrete action plans that consider local needs and context and that, in turn, will increase the support for adoption. Political leadership is key to establish a coherent vision and a strategy for transformation.[33] Local leaders with political skills are essential for implementing change, as they support team performance and manage interorganisational disagreements.[34] The execution of national healthcare action plans requires meticulous project coordination with a proper balance between centralised and decentralised distributed responsibilities.

To accelerate the adoption of digitally enabled, person-centred care, countries must strengthen their capacity to transform their healthcare systems. The core principles of successful Digital Health implementation (i.e., community-based co-creation, service redesign and financial and regulatory alignment) are universal, but their application must be tailored to local contexts and population needs. Additionally, effective change management and a consideration of culture-specific factors are crucial to ensure long-term success.

REFERENCES

1. Gadsby EW, Wilding H. Systems thinking in, and for, public health: a call for a broader path. *Health Promot Int.* 2024;39. https://doi.org/10.1093/heapro/daae086.

2. Cripps M, Scarbrough H. Making digital health 'solutions' sustainable in healthcare systems: a practitioner perspective. *Front Digit Health.* 2022 Mar 31;4:727421. https://doi.org/10.3389/fdgth.2022.727421. PMID: 35434699; PMCID: PMC9008401.

3. Guldemond N. What is meant by 'integrated personalized diabetes management': a view into the future and what success should look like. *Diabetes.* 2024;26:14–29.

4. Guldemond N. *Healthcare as a use case for standardisation in the field of artificial intelligence.* European Commission, Report; 2024 Jul. https://doi.org/10.5281/zenodo.14184600.

5. Steele Gray C, Gagnon D, Guldemond N. Digital health systems in integrated care. In: Amelung V, Stein V, Suter E, et al., editors. *Handbook integrated care.* Cham: Springer; 2021. pp. 479–96. https://doi.org/10.1007/978-3-030-69262-9_28.

6. Khatri RB, Wolka E, Nigatu F, et al. People-centred primary health care: a scoping review. *BMC Prim Care.* 2023;24:236. https://doi.org/10.1186/s12875-023-02194-3.

7. Cunningham S, McNamara S, Cunningham M. Sustainable digital health strategies: navigating long-term success. *J Med Internet Res.* 2022;24(8):e12345. https://doi.org/10.2196/12345.

8. Monaghesh E, Hajizadeh A. The role of telehealth during COVID-19 outbreak: a systematic review based on current evidence. *BMC Public Health.* 2020;20:1193. https://doi.org/10.1186/s12889-020-09301-4.

9. Greenhalgh T, Shaw S, Wherton J, et al. Real-world implementation of video outpatient consultations at macro, meso, and micro levels: mixed-method study. *J Med Internet Res.* 2018;20(4):e150. https://doi.org/10.2196/jmir.9897.

10. Hollis S, Bowie R. Financial sustainability of digital health: strategies and best practices. *J Med Internet Res.* 2021;23(7):e23920. https://doi.org/10.2196/23920.

11. Warren S, Smalley P, Bradshaw M. Evaluating the financial viability of digital health solutions: cost-benefit analyses. *Health Aff (Millwood).* 2020;39(3):455–462. https://doi.org/10.1377/hlthaff.2020.00298.

12. Friedman C, Wyatt JC. *Evaluation methods in biomedical informatics.* 2nd ed. New York: Springer; 2006.

13. García-González J, Agboola SO, Kvedar JC. Scaling digital health interventions: best practices and lessons learned. *JMIR Mhealth Uhealth.* 2021;9(4):e25179. https://doi.org/10.2196/25179.

14. Bradley KL, Shachmut K, Viswanathan S, et al. The role of incentives in health-closing the gap. *Mil Med.* 2018 Nov–Dec;183(Suppl 3):208–12. https://doi.org/10.1093/milmed/usy216.

15. Carlson CJ, Phelan AL. International law reform for one health notifications. *Lancet.* 2022;400:462–68.

16. Franklin B, *One health legislation: contributing to pandemic prevention through law.* Rome: Food and Agriculture Organization of the United Nations; 2020. https://doi.org/10.4060/ca9729en.

17. Destoumieux-Garzón D. The one health concept: 10 years old and a long road ahead. *Front Vet Sci.* 2018;5:14. https://doi.org/10.3389/fvets.2018.00014.

18. Kasse GE, Humphries J, Cosh SM, et al. Factors contributing to the variation in antibiotic prescribing among primary health care physicians: a systematic review. *BMC Prim Care.* 2024;25:8. https://doi.org/10.1186/s12875-023-02223-1.

19. World Health Organization. *Ten threats to global health in 2019.* Available from: https://www.who.int/news-room/spotlight/ten-threats-to-global-health-in-2019.

20. Mohamed A. The synergies between international health regulations and one health in safeguarding global health security. *Sci One Health*. 2024;3:100078. https://doi.org/10.1016/j.soh.2024.100078.

21. Sarkar U, Bates DW. Using artificial intelligence to improve primary care for patients and clinicians. *JAMA Intern Med*. 2024;184(4):343–344. https://doi.org/10.1001/jamainternmed.2023.7965.

22. Kahn SD, Terry SF. Who owns (or controls) health data? *Sci Data*. 2024;11:156. https://doi.org/10.1038/s41597-024-02982-1.

23. General Secretariat of the EU Council. *Analysis of the final compromise text with a view to agreement*. 8571/22 ADD1-8 2022/0140 (COD); 2022. p. 11. Available from: https://www.consilium.europa.eu/media/70909/st07553-en24.pdf.

24. Regulation (EU) 2016/679 of the European Parliament and of the Council, article 4 EU GDPR "Definitions" on the protection of natural persons with regard to the processing of personal data and on the free movement of such data, and repealing Directive 95/46/EC (General Data Protection Regulation); 2016.

25. Proposal for a Regulation of the European Parliament and of the Council on the European Health Data Space, Strasbourg, 2022 May 3, COM(2022) 197 final. 2022/0140 (COD). See Article 8. Available from: https://eur-lex.europa.eu/resource.html?uri=cellar:dbfd8974-cb79-11ec-b6f4-01aa75ed71a1.0001.02/DOC_1&format=PDF.

26. Digital Health Laws and Regulations. *Recent updates on emerging trends in the global regulation of digital health: fragmented frameworks continue striving to catch up with technological advancement 2024–2025*. Available from: https://iclg.com/practice-areas/digital-health-laws-and-regulations.

27. Directive 2011/24/EU of the European Parliament and of the Council of 2011 Mar 9 on the application of patients' rights in cross-border healthcare, article 7(7) 2011. Available from: https://eur-lex.europa.eu/eli/dir/2011/24/oj/eng.

28. Telehealth Regulation. *How is telehealth regulated? Australia*. Available from: https://www.dlapiperintelligence.com/telehealth/countries/index.html?t=02-regulation-of-telehealth&c=AU.

29. Fernandes FA, Chaltikyan GV. Analysis of legal and regulatory frameworks in digital health: a comparison of guidelines and approaches in the European Union and United States. *JISfTeH*. 2020 Dec 14;8(1–3):e11. https://doi.org/10.29086/JISfTeH.8.e11.

30. Purtova N, Kosta E, Koops BJ. Laws and regulations for digital health. In: Fricker S, Thümmler C, Gavras A, editors. *Requirements engineering for digital health*. Cham: Springer; 2015. https://doi.org/10.1007/978-3-319-09798-5_3.

31. Ambrose D. *Managing complex change*. Pittsburgh, PA: The Enterprise Group, Ltd; 1987.

32. Pesapane F, Bracchi DA, Mulligan JF, et al. Legal and regulatory framework for AI solutions in healthcare in EU, US, China, and Russia: new scenarios after a pandemic. *Radiation*. 2021;1:261–76.

33. Clarke JM, Waring J, Bishop S, et al. The contribution of political skill to the implementation of health services change: a systematic review and narrative synthesis. *BMC Health Serv Res*. 2021;21(1):260.

34. NHS. *Improvement—an overview of action planning*. Leicester: National Health Service; 2011. Available from: https://www.england.nhs.uk/improvement-hub/wp-content/uploads/sites/44/2018/06/An-Overview-of-Action-Planning.pdf.

CHAPTER 10

Conclusion

Transforming Primary Care
Through Digital Health

Liliana Laranjo, Sara Ares-Blanco, Amanda Howe, Sankha Randenikumara, and Donald Li

DIGITAL HEALTH FOR PRIMARY CARE: SUMMARY OF KEY INSIGHTS

The integration of Digital Health technologies into Primary Care is rapidly reshaping healthcare delivery. Although there is growing evidence of improved effectiveness, efficiency, safety, patient-centredness, and timeliness of care for some digital tools, equity remains a concern. The COVID-19 pandemic not only led to the accelerated adoption of digital tools to bridge emerging care gaps and enable remote care delivery but also highlighted important barriers to widespread implementation, such as the exacerbation of health inequities due to the digital divide.

Recent developments in artificial intelligence (AI) are showing promise in supporting clinicians and patients in various healthcare tasks, from the automatic documentation of consultations to personalised self-management support. Nevertheless, the evaluation and regulation of these novel technologies are lagging behind their rapid deployment. Rigorous evaluation studies are needed to understand the impact of these novel technologies on the different domains of healthcare quality and their environmental sustainability. This information is key to assisting clinicians, patients, policymakers, and other stakeholders in making evidence-based decisions about their adoption.

FUTURE DIRECTIONS AND EMERGING TRENDS

The future of Digital Health in Primary Care will likely be shaped by rapid technological advancements and evolving healthcare demands. Emerging

DOI: 10.1201/9781003610519-10

trends point to an increased implementation of AI and big data analytics, digital self-management support and patient empowerment, and remote care delivery via telehealth. AI-driven clinical decision support tools that can analyse vast datasets hold the potential to enhance diagnostic accuracy, predict patient outcomes, and support tailored treatment plans.

With the aging of our global population, it is crucial that we understand the challenges and opportunities that lie ahead. The field of gerontology plays a vital role in shaping policies, developing innovative solutions, and fostering a society that values and supports older adults. Innovation and technology have the potential to revolutionise the way that we approach aging. From advancements in medical research to smart home technologies and telehealth, we have an unprecedented opportunity to enhance the lives of older adults. It is our duty to leverage these tools and ensure that they are accessible to all, regardless of socioeconomic status or geographical location.

Telehealth is poised to evolve further by integrating advanced technologies such as real-time language translation, remote diagnostics, and remote health monitoring with wearable devices. These innovations hold the potential to enhance access and convenience, especially for populations in rural or underserved regions. At the same time, additional AI developments will support the scale-up of mobile technology interventions that can deliver personalised education and behaviour change support to chronic disease patients in their preferred language.

Addressing Digital Health inequities remains a critical focus. Efforts to bridge the digital divide must include initiatives to improve digital literacy, expand internet access, and subsidise technologies for marginalised communities. As hybrid care models that combine digital and in-person care delivery gain traction, there is a growing emphasis on establishing guidelines to balance innovation with patient-centred principles and equity. Sustainability is another emerging priority, with calls for environmentally friendly Digital Health solutions that reduce healthcare's carbon footprint.

Collaboration among stakeholders—policymakers, healthcare providers, researchers, technology developers, and patients—will be key to shaping a future where Digital Health augments rather than replaces traditional care. Research into the short- and long-term impacts of these digital tectonic shifts is crucial to avoid unintended consequences and to ensure improvements in all domains of quality of care.

RECOMMENDATIONS FOR PRIMARY CARE PROVIDERS AND POLICYMAKERS

In light of the growing evidence that the new digital technology era can enhance the quality of Primary Care delivery,[1] it is important to address several key recommendations for providers, training organisations, and policymakers to ensure effective implementation.

First, ensuring that the necessary infrastructure and technical expertise are in place is key for the successful implementation of Digital Health initiatives in Primary Care. Adequate technology infrastructure is context-dependent but should include relevant hardware (e.g., computers), internet access, and interoperable software tools that guarantee data privacy and security. Maintaining and improving the existing technology infrastructure will also require staff who possess the skills and technical expertise to select, install, maintain, and evaluate these systems and to train others in their use. Readily available technical support is paramount to supporting clinicians when system failures occur, as daily clinical practice becomes more reliant on electronic medical records. Therefore, the allocation of adequate resources and investment is key to supporting and enhancing Digital Health transformation in modern Primary Care services.

Training is another critical area of focus.[2] Comprehensive training programs tailored to staff roles and responsibilities are imperative to ensuring that everyone can use existing and new technologies effectively. Induction programs for new team members and ongoing audits of system usage are necessary to maintain safe and consistent practices. Specific staff, such as nurses assisting patients with self-monitoring devices, may require additional personalised training to address patients' unique needs.

Digital transformation efforts in Primary Care must be strategically planned and standardised across providers in a given region. Standard operating procedures for the use of electronic medical records, digital tools, and electronic communication should be co-designed and implemented with Primary Care providers. Providers must also develop and follow localised procedures for determining which clinical work can safely be conducted remotely through email, phone, or video interactions. These strategies should address how to maintain continuity of care across remote and in-person encounters. Similarly, protocols for digitally enhanced integrated care are essential, particularly for identifying patients suitable for remote referrals to other clinicians (e.g., specialists and allied health services). Such protocols can reduce patient travel and lower out-of-pocket expenses and the travel-related carbon footprint.

Providers can also leverage technology to enhance patient-centred care. User-friendly organisational websites can support patients by detailing available services and offering secure patient access for appointments, prescriptions, clinical queries, and medical record viewing.[3] Online systems can further be leveraged to support patient education and provide reliable health information and resources. Importantly, Primary Care providers should actively address barriers to patient use of implemented technologies to avoid further inequities because of the digital divide. Ensuring routine patient feedback on digital services is essential for quality improvement.

Organisations that train Primary Care providers have additional responsibilities. They should develop relevant curricula and learning opportunities to equip future doctors, nurses, and managers with the skills to effectively utilise modern digital technologies. Sharing knowledge through professional meetings and continuing professional development events, both online and in person, is critical for continuously developing capacity in Primary Care Digital Health. Guidance should also be provided to help providers develop and adopt appropriate standard operating procedures for choosing and using different technologies.

Policymakers play a crucial role in shaping the broader digital transformation of Primary Care. They must plan and implement strategies that ensure system-wide delivery of training, infrastructure, and evidence-based Digital Health solutions that are safe and effective. Coordinating these strategies at the system level helps ensure consistency and equity.

Policymakers should also invest in national evidence-building and research that evaluates the impact of Digital Health interventions, such as emerging AI tools, on health and patient-reported outcomes, care efficiency, equity, and patient and staff experience based on the quintuple aim framework.[4]

Ultimately, the health sector's approach to digital technology is more effective when coordinated at the government and national levels rather than when it is driven by individual providers or commercial interests. A unified strategy ensures that digital innovations benefit all stakeholders and foster a more equitable and efficient healthcare system.

POLICY IMPLICATIONS AND HEALTHCARE REFORM

The implementation of Digital Health in Primary Care should follow a shared long-term vision for health reform that aims to improve health and patient outcomes, care efficiency, equity, patient and workforce experience, and environmental sustainability. Health reform can be defined as "the purposeful use of policy options to effect changes that are intended to improve the performance of the health system".[5] A health reform centred on Digital Health for Primary Care should ideally follow a systematic and strategic approach for successful health system strengthening. First, a comprehensive review of the key components of the healthcare system should be performed to identify performance gaps and their causes. Next, the status of Digital Health within the country or region should be assessed by reviewing the availability, adoption, and integration of digital tools in the existing healthcare system to pinpoint the gaps and areas for improvement. Understanding the baseline allows for a targeted and effective reform strategy. Updated legislation and government policies should be sought before implementing the reform and may include researching and keeping track of recent legislative changes, proposals, and discussions within government bodies, studying best practices, and looking at successful reforms in other regions or countries for guidance. Furthermore, there should be advocacy for legislative support that builds coalitions and forms alliances with organisations that share similar goals to strengthen advocacy efforts.

Identifying and engaging all stakeholders is a vital component of the reform process. Healthcare professionals, patients, technology experts, policymakers, and industry should all be included in discussions to ensure that the reform addresses the population's needs and priorities. Clear objectives and implementation timelines for policies must be defined with all stakeholders to guide the reform process. It is key to consider the diverse socioeconomic strata of the population to design a reform that is feasible and equitable. This dialogue ensures that the reform is practical, widely accepted, and aligned with the healthcare ecosystem's realities and challenges.[6]

Patient engagement and empowerment are critical, requiring strategies to educate the population about digital tools such as health-tracking apps, medical records, and appointment scheduling. It is important to address the digital divide and digital literacy, with simplified processes designed for patients unfamiliar with technology, to ensure equitable access. Patients should be enabled to easily book remote consultations, with a focus on promoting this option for straightforward cases involving low-comorbidity patients. Additionally, pilot projects of remote consultations for chronic disease management can help identify the conditions that would benefit most from this approach.

Healthcare budgeting and resource allocation are fundamental to the success of the reform. This includes understanding the technical requirements, such as infrastructure, hardware, and software, and safeguarding secure access to these tools with reliable connectivity across all health centres. When implementing such reforms, it is recommended for IT services to be interoperable across regions within the same country and, if possible, internationally. The World Health Organization (WHO) has evaluated Primary Care information systems in the European region and developed a strategy for their optimisation; it is therefore recommended to follow this guidance when designing such systems.

The financial impact on both patients and healthcare professionals must be carefully assessed, with adequate regulations in place to support these changes. To ensure effective future financial planning, it is crucial to clearly identify and engage all relevant stakeholders, including private enterprises, potential investors, and public-private cooperative ventures. These entities play key roles in providing the necessary resources, expertise, and funding to support the implementation and sustainability of reforms, particularly in areas such as Digital Health and Primary Care innovation. Long-term financial planning should consider team salaries, operational costs, potential consultancy needs, contracting mechanisms, and overall funding sources to sustain the reform. Mechanisms should also be put in place to ensure transparency, accountability, and the equitable sharing of financial and operational risks. Additionally, the cost of the reform should not be directly passed to patients or self-employed healthcare professionals. Thus, a government plan with state funding is necessary to modernise information systems and telehealth platforms.

Continuous evaluation and monitoring are necessary to measure the reform's effectiveness across key dimensions. These include health outcomes, such as improvements in population health, care efficiency, equity, and patient satisfaction. Additionally, the reform should aim to reduce the administrative burden on General Practitioners, alleviating workload and work-related stress and burnout through the use of Digital Health. It is essential to evaluate the usability of the technology and the time required for it to connect properly. Time is one of the most valuable resources in Primary Care consultations, so it is necessary for professionals to know in advance how much time the tool requires to be used effectively, without impacting the time dedicated to patient care. Key building blocks of high-performing Primary Care should also be monitored, including data-driven improvement, team-based care, prompt access to care, continuity of care, and care coordination.[7] It is important to continuously evaluate the implementation of health policies and monitor the process and outcome measures compared with traditional care to ensure that Digital Health innovations are used where they are proven to be most beneficial.

A NEW VISION FOR THE FUTURE OF PRIMARY CARE

Digital Health offers unparalleled opportunities to enhance the quality of Primary Care delivery globally. Realising these benefits will likely require a balanced approach to health reform and policies that embrace a hybrid model of care which synergistically combines the strengths of digital tools with the irreplaceable value of face-to-face interactions while investing in inclusive infrastructure and policy frameworks.

The effective integration of Digital Health requires addressing safety, equity, and usability concerns through collaborative, evidence-based strategies that ensure these tools complement rather than disrupt the patient-physician relationship. Patient empowerment through tools such as personal health records and educational resources is central to this transformation, fostering shared decision-making and proactive health management.

Policymakers must prioritise establishing regulatory frameworks that safeguard patient safety, data privacy, and equity while promoting innovation.

Collaborative efforts among stakeholders will be essential to develop ethical, user-friendly, and sustainable Digital Health solutions. Investments in education, training, and support for healthcare providers are crucial to equip them with the skills needed to navigate the digital landscape effectively and prevent burnout.

Looking ahead, the vision for Primary Care extends beyond technology integration to encompass a systemic approach to healthcare delivery. This includes fostering multidisciplinary collaborations, strengthening community health networks, and adopting value-based care models that prioritise outcomes over volume. By aligning Digital Health innovations with these broader goals, Primary Care can evolve into a more resilient and responsive system capable of meeting the challenges of a dynamic healthcare landscape.

Ultimately, the future of Primary Care lies in striking a balance between technological progress and the enduring values of trust, compassion, and equity that define the patient-physician relationship. With thoughtful planning and inclusive strategies, Digital Health can serve as a catalyst for achieving a healthcare system that is not only technologically advanced but also deeply human-centric.

KEY MESSAGES

- Hybrid, digitally enabled models of care can combine the strengths of digital tools with the irreplaceable value of face-to-face interactions to augment Primary Care delivery.
- The transformation of Primary Care into high-functioning digitally enabled systems will require strategic health reform with careful consideration of infrastructure, population needs, workforce training, funding and resource allocation.
- The continuous evaluation and monitoring of digital transformation in Primary Care is needed to ensure that the benefits of quality of care always outweigh any potential harms and unintended consequences.

REFERENCES

1. World Health Organization. *Digital technologies: shaping the future of primary health care*. Geneva: World Health Organization; 2018.
2. Jimenez G, Spinazze P, Matchar D, et al. Digital health competencies for primary healthcare professionals: a scoping review. *Int J Med Inform*. 2020 Nov 1;143:104260.
3. Benjamins J, Haveman-Nies A, Gunnink M, et al. How the use of a patient-accessible health record contributes to patient-centered care: scoping review. *J Med Internet Res*. 2021 Jan 11;23(1):e17655.

4. Nundy S, Cooper LA, Mate KS. The quintuple aim for health care improvement: a new imperative to advance health equity. *JAMA*. 2022 Feb 8;327(6):521–2.

5. Reich MR, Campos PA, Kalita A, et al. *Guide to health reform: eight practical steps.* Boston: Harvard T. H. Chan School of Public Health; 2023.

6. Williams S, Barnard A, Collis P, et al. Remote consultations in primary care across low-, middle-and high-income countries: implications for policy and care delivery. *J Health Serv Res Policy*. 2023 Jul;28(3):181–9.

7. Bodenheimer T, Ghorob A, Willard-Grace R, et al. The 10 building blocks of high-performing primary care. *Ann Fam Med*. 2014 Mar 1;12(2):166–71.

Index

Note: Page numbers in *italics* indicate a figure and page numbers in **bold** indicate a table on the corresponding page.